Poc

Veterinary Nurses

Editor:

Louise O'Dwyer
MBA BSc(Hons) VTS(ECC)
DipAVN(Medical & Surgical) RVN

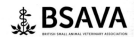

BSAVA
BRITISH SMALL ANIMAL VETERINARY ASSOCIATION

Published by:
British Small Animal Veterinary Association
Woodrow House, 1 Telford Way, Waterwells Business Park,
Quedgeley, Gloucester GL2 2AB

A Company Limited by Guarantee in England.
Registered Company No. 2837793.
Registered as a Charity.

First published 2013
Reprinted 2015, 2016, 2017, 2018, 2019
Copyright © 2019 BSAVA

Illustrations showing direct blood pressure measurement, blood
smear preparation, arterial blood sampling, venous blood sampling,
Robert Jones bandage, ear and head bandage, thoracic bandage,
abdominal bandage, foot and lower limb bandage, Velpeau sling,
Ehmer sling, tail bandage, cross-matching and advanced
radiographic positioning were drawn by S.J. Elmhurst BA Hons
(www.livingart.org.uk) and are printed with her permission.

Illustrations showing basic radiographic positioning were drawn by
Charlotte Nagle and are printed with her permission.

Stock photography: © Monika Wisniewska | Dreamstime.com

A catalogue record for this book is available from the British Library.

ISBN 978-1-905319-52-7

The publishers, editors and contributors cannot take responsibility for
information provided on dosages and methods of application of
drugs mentioned or referred to in this publication. Details of this kind
must be verified in each case by individual users from up to date
literature published by the manufacturers or suppliers of those drugs.
Veterinary surgeons are reminded that in each case they must follow
all appropriate national legislation and regulations (for example, in the
United Kingdom, the prescribing cascade) from time to time in force.

Printed in the UK by Zenith Media, Cardiff
Printed on ECF paper made from sustainable forests

7922PUBS19

Contents

■ Foreword   v
■ Preface   vi
■ A few notes on using this book   vii

■ Part 1: Patient assessment
  – Normal range of vital signs in commonly seen species   1
  – Routine patient parameter assessments   2
  – Daily tasks   2
  – Mucous membrane colour   5
  – Pain assessment   6
  – Nutritional assessment   7
  – Body Condition System for dogs   8
  – Body Condition System for cats   10
  – Blood pressure measurement   12
  – Blood pressure values for dogs and cats   16
  – How to obtain an electrocardiogram   16

■ Part 2: Inpatient care
  – Recumbent patients   21
  – Intravenous catheter management   22
  – Cleaning urinary catheters   22
  – Selection of feeding tubes   23
  – Calculating resting energy requirement (RER)   23
  – Nursing considerations for feeding tubes   24
  – Physiotherapy   24

■ Part 3: Laboratory
  – Blood   31
  – Urine   44
  – Common faecal examinations   45
  – Hair and skin sampling procedures   46
  – Fine needle aspiration of a mass   51
  – Packaging laboratory samples for external analysis   53

➡

■ **Part 4: Bandaging and wound care**

- Wound dressings   57
- Robert Jones bandage   62
- Ear and head bandage   64
- Thoracic bandage   65
- Abdominal bandage   66
- Foot and lower limb bandage   67
- Velpeau sling   68
- Ehmer sling   69
- Tail bandage   70
- Management of wound drains   71

■ **Part 5: Triage and emergency care**

- Fluid therapy   75
- Blood transfusion   79

■ **Part 6: Imaging**

- Radiographic positioning   97
- Advanced radiographic positioning   119
- Film faults   125

■ **Part 7: Anaesthesia and analgesia**

- ASA scale of anaesthetic risk   129
- Anaesthetic equipment   130
- Drugs   144
- Anaesthetic emergencies   150

■ **Part 8: Theatre**

- Cleaning and sterilization   155
- Gowning and gloving   162
- Scrubbing   167
- Sutures   170

■ **References**   **177**
■ **Index**   **178**
■ **Emergency doses for dogs and cats**   **184**

Foreword

I am honoured to have been asked to write the Foreword for the first edition of the *BSAVA Pocketbook for Veterinary Nurses*.

Veterinary nurses are now an integral part of the Practice Team. Their responsibilities and knowledge have grown rapidly over the years and this is reflected in the amount of information in the *BSAVA Textbook of Veterinary Nursing, 5th Edition*.

Nurses, however, need to be able to access some of this information concisely and accurately in a book they can carry around in their pocket. This pocketbook fills that need. It is packed with information on the important techniques that are part of the day-to-day work of the veterinary nurse, from pain assessment to blood pressure measurement. The illustrations are excellent and the wording clear and concise.

The team behind this publication has produced an exceptional guide that allows very rapid access to information and saves that most important commodity for nurses – time.

This pocketbook is thus yet another good reason for nurses to join BSAVA.

Mark R. Johnston
BVetMed MRCVS

BSAVA President 2012–13

Preface

The BSAVA Pocketbook for Nurses is a new initiative from the Membership Development Committee of the BSAVA in response to feedback from members. The book has been designed as a 'quick reference' guide, providing a range of essential and useful information easily at hand. Many of us carried around homemade 'pocketbooks' during our training (and possibly still do) and my aim was to put together this information in a concise format that nurses, whether training or qualified, can easily refer to. This book does not replace any of the existing BSAVA nursing manuals but instead is designed to complement them. Provision has also been made to allow nurses to make their own additional notes for completeness.

I would like to thank Michelle Stead, chair of the Membership Development Committee, and the publishing team at BSAVA for their help and guidance when preparing this pocketbook. I would also like to thank and acknowledge the huge number of BSAVA authors whose work I have harvested from other Manuals and articles for inclusion here. Without these people this book could not exist.

Finally, as this is the first edition and a new venture, I would welcome suggestions for inclusion (and teething problems for exclusion!) in future editions. Please contact me via **publications@bsava.com,** putting VN Pocketbook in the subject line.

Louise O'Dwyer
MBA BSc(Hons) VTS(ECC) DipAVN(Medical & Surgical) RVN

December 2012

A few notes on using this book

- This book is designed to condense the common nursing procedures into one pocket-sized book that can be carried around easily in a tunic or scrub top pocket.
- It contains much of the basic information on certain procedures; for more detailed information a more in-depth text should be consulted.
- All procedures should be carried out under the direction of a veterinary surgeon; veterinary nurses should ensure they carry out these procedures under the remit of Schedule 3 of the Veterinary Surgeons Act 1966 (Part 1, paragraphs 6 and 7).
- Selected drugs are listed by generic name.
- All medications should be administered under the direction of a veterinary surgeon.
- A veterinary nurse should always refer to other source material if they are not familiar with the procedures mentioned in this guide.

Patient assessment

Normal range of vital signs in commonly seen species[9]

Species	Body temperature (°C)	Heart rate (beats/min)	Respiratory rate (breaths/min)
Dog	38.3–39.2	70–140	10–30
Cat	38.2–38.6	100–200	20–30
Ferret	37.8–40	200–250	33–36
Domestic rabbit	38.5–40	130–325	30–60
Chinchilla	37–38	200–350	40–80
Guinea pig	37.2–39.5	230–380	90–150
Chipmunk	38 (during torpor, a few degrees above ambient)	264–296 (during torpor, may drop to 3–6)	75 (during torpor, may drop to <1 and is barely detectable)
Gerbil	37.4–39	260–600	85–160
Hamster (Russian)	36–38	300–460	60–80
Hamster (Syrian)	36.2–37.5	300–470	40–110
Rat	38	310–500	70–150
Mouse	37.5	420–700	100–250

Routine patient parameter assessments[2]

Body system/ assessment	Parameter	Intervals
Cardiovascular	Pulse rate and quality Mucous membranes Capillary refill time Arterial blood pressure Central venous pressure (if central catheter present)	Every 1–6 h
Respiratory	Respiratory rate and effort Oxygen saturation (pulse oximeter)	Every 1–6 h
Demeanour	Patient appearance and behaviour	Every 2–6 h
Temperature		Every 2–12 h
Urination assessment	Walk, check tray, check bladder and drain urinary collection bag Calculate ml/kg/h and specific gravity when obtainable	Every 2–4 h
Wounds/ dressings/ intravenous catheters	Tension, swelling and discharge	Every 4–12 h
Intravenous catheters	Flush	Every 4 h
Arterial catheters	Flush	Every 1 h
Recumbent patients	Ensure patient is turned	At least every 4 h

Daily tasks[9]

- **Record temperature, pulse and respiration (TPR).**
  These essential parameters should be recorded while the patient is in a calm state (prior to exercise) in order to obtain accurate measurements.

- **Record bodyweight.** This will highlight any changes during the period of hospitalization, possibly due to anorexia or fluid accumulation.
- **Evaluate mental state** of the patient. Is the animal bright, responsive, disoriented, depressed, etc.? These subjective findings can help to determine whether a patient is progressing or deteriorating.
- **Opportunity to exercise and eliminate outside the kennel.** Dogs should be taken outside 3–4 times daily if appropriate; other patients should be provided with litter trays or areas of the kennel that are away from the bedding area.
- **Observation of wounds** should be performed at least once daily for signs of swelling, discharge, dehiscence, or interference. Dressings or bandages should be changed as necessary.
- **Monitoring for signs of pain or discomfort** should be performed continuously throughout the day and the clinician informed of any change in the patient's condition.
- **Medication** should be administered at the appropriate times and in the correct way.
- **Provide nutritional requirements** (unless nil per mouth). The correct food should be provided and a record kept specifying what food has been offered and the quantity consumed.
- **Correct care of intravenous catheters.** Peripheral intravenous catheters should be flushed twice daily to ensure patency, and insertion sites inspected for signs of contamination. Catheters should be removed and replaced in another location if necessary.
- **Appropriate care of wound or cavity drains and feeding tubes.** Insertion sites should be checked at least twice daily and bandaged as necessary. Draining fluids should be recorded.
- **Maintain patient hygiene.** All patients should be examined for areas of soiling of their coats, and bathed and groomed as necessary.
- **Physiotherapy** – should be performed on recumbent or inactive patients, usually 2–4 times daily.

NOTES

Mucous membrane colour[9]

- **Pale** membranes are indicative of poor perfusion; this may be seen in patients with circulatory collapse, haemorrhage, anaemia or severe vasoconstriction.
- **Red** ('congested') membranes may indicate sepsis, fever, congestion, causes of extensive tissue damage or excitement.
- **Blue or purple** membranes (cyanosis) indicate severe hypoxaemia (lack of oxygen in the blood); this could be caused by respiratory difficulty, and immediate action must be taken to increase the patient's oxygen saturation.
- **Yellow** membranes (icterus/jaundice) may be due to liver disease, bile flow obstruction or an increase in red blood cell destruction and circulating bilirubin.
- **Orange** membranes may be seen after administration of synthetic haemoglobin products.
- **Chocolate brown** mucous membranes in dogs and cats are indicative of paracetamol poisoning. Cats are unable to metabolize paracetamol, and toxicity therefore occurs after consumption of even low doses.
- **Cherry red** membranes are seen in patients suffering from carbon monoxide poisoning, for example as a result of exposure to car exhaust or fire fumes.

NOTES

Pain assessment[3]

Key points

- Assume that humans and animals are closely similar in terms of pain perception and anticipation, and manage pain accordingly.
- At present, response to appropriate analgesia remains the best marker for accurate diagnosis of pain.
- Remember that breed, age, illness, temperament and drug administration influence behavioural responses to pain.
- Since the pain experience can alter rapidly, pain assessment must be performed frequently.
- Pain assessors should have experience in pain assessment and be familiar with the patient.
- Compare an animal's behaviour before and after the onset of pain where this is possible (i.e. pre- and postoperatively), so that improvement or deterioration can be evaluated realistically.
- Assess response to interaction with a handler in addition to simple observation in the cage.
- Assess response to gentle palpation or manipulation of the affected area.
- Look for subtle indicators of pain, particularly in sick patients. Remember that invasive procedures, trauma and medical illnesses cause pain, and may leave animals unable to demonstrate explicit pain behaviour. Certain animals may respond to pain through withdrawal.
- Develop clinic protocols for assessment of acute and chronic pain. An ideal scoring system should be relatively easy to use by all staff, with clearly defined assessment criteria, and validated in a clinical setting.
- Reassess. Re-evaluate analgesic efficacy. Re-administer analgesia appropriately as assessment requires.

Behavioural indicators of pain

- Dog
  - Hyperalgesia or allodynia
  - Postures: hunching, 'praying', not resting in a normal position

- Locomotion: stiff, no weightbearing on affected limb
- Vocalization: barking, growling, whining
- Facial expressions: ear position, eye position
- Attention to (or guarding of) the affected area
- Aggression
- Inappetence
- Weak tail wag

■ Cat
- *As for dog, with additionally:*
- Vocalization: hissing
- Facial expressions: furrowed brow, ears pinned back
- Depression, no self-grooming
- Hunched immobile stance
- Hyperventilation
- Ears pulled back
- Sitting in back of cage or hiding under blanket
- Pupillary dilation
- Restlessness
- Tachypnoea or panting

Pain scales

■ Visual analogue scale (VAS)
■ Numerical rating scale (NRS)
■ Simple descriptive scale (SDS)
■ Composite scoring system
■ Multidimensional scoring system

Nutritional assessment[8]

The Nestlé Purina Body Condition Systems for Dogs and Cats are illustrated on the following pages. Other body condition scoring systems exist, such as the Waltham® S.H.A.P.E.™ Guide for Dogs and the Waltham® S.H.A.P.E.™ Guide for Cats. ➡

▦ Nestlé PURINA
Body Condition System for dogs

TOO THIN

1 Ribs, lumbar vertebrae, pelvic bones and all bony prominences evident from a distance. No discernible body fat. Obvious loss of muscle mass.

2 Ribs, lumbar vertebrae and pelvic bones easily visible. No palpable fat. Some evidence of other bony prominence. Minimal loss of muscle mass.

3 Ribs easily palpated and may be visible with no palpable fat. Tops of lumbar vertebrae visible. Pelvic bones becoming prominent. Obvious waist and abdominal tuck.

IDEAL

4 Ribs easily palpable, with minimal fat covering. Waist easily noted, viewed from above. Abdominal tuck evident.

5 Ribs palpable without excess fat covering. Waist observed behind ribs when viewed from above. Abdomen tucked up when viewed from side.

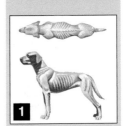

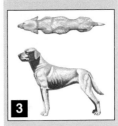

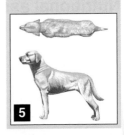

TOO HEAVY

6 Ribs palpable with slight excess fat covering. Waist is discernible viewed from above but is not prominent. Abdominal tuck apparent.

7 Ribs palpable with difficulty; heavy fat cover. Noticeable fat deposits over lumbar area and base of tail. Waist absent or barely visible. Abdominal tuck may be present.

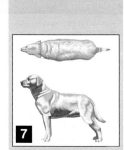

8 Ribs not palpable under very heavy fat cover, or palpable only with significant pressure. Heavy fat deposits over lumbar area and base of tail. Waist absent. No abdominal tuck. Obvious abdominal distention may be present.

9 Massive fat deposits over thorax, spine and base of tail. Waist and abdominal tuck absent. Fat deposits on neck and limbs. Obvious abdominal distention.

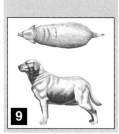

9-point body condition scale for dogs. (© Nestlé Purina PetCare and reproduced with their permission.)

The BODY CONDITION SYSTEM was developed at the Nestlé Purina Pet Care Center and has been validated as documented in the following publications:

Mawby D, Bartges JW, Moyers T, *et. al.* **Comparison of body fat estimates by dual-energy x-ray absorptiometry and deuterium oxide dilution in client owned dogs.** Compendium 2001; 23 (9A): 70

Laflamme DP. **Development and Validation of a Body Condition Score System for Dogs.** Canine Practice July/August 1997; 22: 10–15

Kealy, *et. al.* **Effects of Diet Restriction on Life Span and Age-Related Changes in Dogs.** JAVMA 2002; 220: 1315–1320

➡

▦ Nestlé PURINA
Body Condition System for cats

TOO THIN

1 Ribs visible on shorthaired cats; no palpable fat; severe abdominal tuck; lumbar vertebrae and wings of ilia easily palpated.

2 Ribs easily visible on shorthaired cats; lumbar vertebrae obvious with minimal muscle mass; pronounced abdominal tuck; no palpable fat.

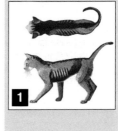

3 Ribs easily palpable with minimal fat covering; lumbar vertebrae obvious; obvious waist behind ribs; minimal abdominal fat.

4 Ribs palpable with minimal fat covering; noticeable waist behind ribs; slight abdominal tuck; abdominal fat pad absent.

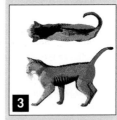

IDEAL

5 Well-proportioned; observe waist behind ribs; ribs palpable with slight fat covering; abdominal fat pad minimal.

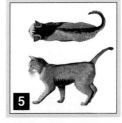

TOO HEAVY

6 Ribs palpable with slight excess fat covering; waist and abdominal fat pad distinguishable but not obvious; abdominal tuck absent.

7 Ribs not easily palpated with moderate fat covering; waist poorly discernible; obvious rounding of abdomen; moderate abdominal fat pad.

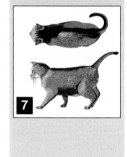

8 Ribs not palpable with excess fat covering; waist absent; obvious rounding of abdomen with prominent abdominal fat pad; fat deposits present over lumbar area.

9 Ribs not palpable under heavy fat cover; heavy fat deposits over lumbar area, face and limbs; distention of abdomen with no waist; extensive abdominal fat deposits.

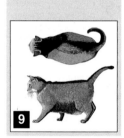

9-point body condition scale for cats. (© Nestlé Purina PetCare and reproduced with their permission.)

Blood pressure measurement[1]

Direct blood pressure measurement

Indications/Use

- Monitoring arterial blood pressure in critically ill patients
- Monitoring arterial blood pressure during anaesthesia
- *Arterial catheters can also be used for serial collection of arterial blood samples for blood gas analysis in animals with pulmonary disease*

Contraindications

- Coagulopathy: arterial catheters may be placed but only with care and only into distal limb arteries
- Arterial catheters should not be placed at sites where risk of bacterial contamination and infection are high, e.g. due to local tissue damage, local skin infection, diarrhoea, urinary incontinence

Indirect blood pressure measurement

Non-invasive blood pressure measurements are technically less demanding than invasive measurements and can be rapidly applied in the emergency situation, although they might not fulfil the expectations of reliability and accuracy. There are two non-invasive methods in general use: the oscillometric method and the Doppler method. Both require a cuff.

Indications/Use

- To assess cardiovascular function
- Routine monitoring during anaesthesia

Equipment

- Doppler ultrasound probe
- Coupling gel
- Adhesive tape
- Inflatable cuff attached to a manometer
  OR
- Oscillometric blood pressure monitor with cuffs

The proper cuff width is 40% of the circumference of the site where the cuff will be placed. Cuffs that are too wide lead to falsely low readings; those that are too narrow lead to falsely high readings.

Patient preparation and positioning

- Can be performed on conscious, sedated or anaesthetized animals.

   Assessment of general cardiovascular status should be made in the absence of sedative and anaesthetic drugs.

- For conscious animals, it is important that they are relaxed and that the limb used is not weight-bearing. Lateral recumbency, with the limb to be used uppermost, is often preferred.
- For the Doppler technique it is necessary to shave the appropriate site and apply adequate coupling gel.

Technique

Doppler ultrasound

An inflatable cuff attached to a manometer occludes an artery, and a piezoelectric crystal placed over the artery distal to the cuff detects flow. The re-entry of blood into the artery as the cuff is released causes a frequency change (Doppler shift) in sound waves, which is detected by the piezoelectric crystal and converted to a sound detected by the operator. **This method measures systolic pressure.**

1. Position the Doppler ultrasound probe over one of the following:
   - The palmar arterial arch, on the ventral aspect of the proximal metacarpal region
   - The plantar arterial arch, on the ventral aspect of the proximal metatarsal region
   - The median caudal artery on the ventral aspect of the tail.

➡

2. Apply coupling gel directly to the transducer and position it so that the sound of flow is detected. Tape the transducer in place perpendicular to the artery.
3. Place the cuff around the limb proximal to the measurement site, avoiding the joints, or around the tail. The cuff should be applied snugly enough to allow insertion of only a small finger between the cuff and the leg or tail. Most cuffs have a mark that should be placed directly over the artery.

> If the cuff is applied too tightly, the measurement will be erroneously low because the cuff partly occludes the artery; if applied too loosely, the measurement will be erroneously high because excessive cuff pressure will be required to occlude the artery.

The cuff must be prevented from moving down the leg or tail when inflated, either by flexing the carpus or tarsus, or by blocking distal movement of the cuff by placing a hand on the appendage, not on the cuff.
4. Inflate the cuff to a pressure above the expected systolic pressure to occlude the artery. This will result in loss of the sound of flow.
5. Slowly deflate the cuff by a few mmHg per second until the sound of flow is again detected. At this time the cuff pressure is equal to the systolic pressure. In patients with very low systolic blood pressure (<70 mmHg), the value obtained may be closer to the mean rather than the systolic pressure.

Oscillometric technique

This uses a cuff to occlude the artery, and detects oscillations of the underlying artery when it is partly occluded. **This system determines systolic, diastolic and mean arterial pressures.** This method is less accurate in very small patients, patients with low blood pressure and patients with arrhythmias. Muscle contractions also create oscillations and are a source of potential error.

1. Place the cuff snugly (see Step 3 above) over one of the following:
   - The radial artery proximal to the carpus
   - The saphenous artery proximal to the tarsus
   - The brachial artery proximal to the elbow
   - The median caudal artery at the base of the tail.
2. Attach the cuff to a control unit that continually senses arterial pressure and inflates to a pressure greater than systolic, and then automatically deflates the cuff.
3. The heart rate is displayed; verify that it matches the patient's heart rate by manually counting the heart rate by direct heart auscultation or palpation of an artery.
4. Record the values for 3–5 cycles and report the averages for systolic, diastolic and mean pressures.

Potential false readings

Incorrect blood pressure readings may be obtained due to:

- Inappropriate cuff size
- Inappropriate placement of the cuff
- Excessive motion of the limb or tail
- Low blood pressure
- Arrhythmias
- Obesity
- Peripheral oedema
- Limb conformation that does not permit snug placement of the cuff
- Stress.

NOTES

Blood pressure values for dogs and cats[4,5]

Blood pressure classification	Systolic BP (mmHg)	Diastolic BP (mmHg)
Hypotension	<90	<50
Normal	Dog: 110–190 Cat: 120–170	Dog: 55–100 Cat: 70–120
Minimal risk of hypertensive TOD	<150	<95
Mild risk of hypertensive TOD	150–159	95–99
Moderate risk of hypertensive TOD	160–179	100–119
Severe risk of hypertensive TOD	>180	>120

TOD = target organ damage

How to obtain an electrocardiogram[2]

1. Place patient on a dry insulated surface.
2. Use standard positioning if this is not too distressing for the patient.
3. Attach one electrode on each limb in the standard configuration (Einthoven's limb lead system): on the forelimbs just above or below the olecranon; and on the hindlimbs just above or below the stifle. Electrodes can be stainless steel crocodile clips or adhesive patches (adhesive patch electrodes are best for long-term monitoring). Electrode jelly is used with clips to improve skin contact. Surgical spirit may be used but needs regular application as it evaporates.

   ■ Red lead – right forelimb.
   ■ Yellow lead – left forelimb.
   ■ Green lead – left hindlimb.
   ■ Black lead – right hindlimb.

Do not allow the electrodes to contact each other. Keep the patient as still as possible during the procedure.

4. Record 5–10 complexes of leads I, II, III, aVr, aVl and aVf at paper speed 25 mm/second.
5. Record a rhythm strip of lead II at paper speed 50 mm/second.
6. Run a longer rhythm strip at a slower speed if possible when checking for dysrhythmia.
7. Record patient details, date, position and any drugs administered for reference.
8. Make a note of the paper speed, calibration (cm:mV) and whether filters were used.

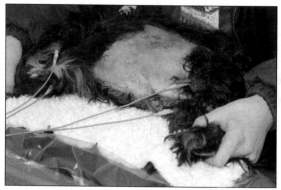

Standard positioning for a diagnostic ECG. The dog is restrained in right lateral recumbency with the limbs extended.

NOTES

NOTES

NOTES

NOTES

PART 2

Inpatient care

Recumbent patients[2]

Actual problems	Potential problems	Nursing plan
Inability to mobilize	Decubitus ulcers, hypostatic pneumonia, stiff joints, muscle contracture	Assisted walking, coupage, turning, padded non-retentive bedding, physiotherapy
Tachypnoea, restlessness or discomfort	Hyperthermia	Regular assessment of analgesic requirements
Loss of voluntary urination or incontinence	Bladder atony, urine scald	Bladder management: indwelling urinary catheter or assist patient outside for urination; use non-retentive bedding
Inability to eat and drink unaided or unable to reach food	Dehydration, poor nutrition leading to delayed healing	Tempt, hand-feed, encourage fluid intake, intravenous fluid therapy, record food intake, consider tube feeding
Inability to maintain body temperature	Hypothermia, thermal burns from inappropriate warming techniques	Patient warming (warm air) and temperature monitoring
Inability to groom and clean	Matted coat, pyoderma	Daily grooming/bath

Intravenous catheter management[2,9]

- Management must be exemplary, as many critically ill patients are immunosuppressed and likely to contract infections easily.
- Washing of hands is mandatory and wearing of gloves advisable. Ensure aseptic handling of the catheter at all times.
- Clean any spilt blood from around the catheter with antiseptic solution, and ensure that all tapes securing catheters and dressings are clean.
- Maintain catheter patency by flushing with heparinized saline (4 units of heparin per 1 ml of 0.9% saline) every 4–6 hours.
- Change peripheral catheters regularly (usually every 3–5 days), in line with instructions from the veterinary surgeon in charge. Jugular lines are rarely changed if they are functioning well.
- Inspect the skin insertion site of jugular catheters at least three times daily, with gloved hands. Check for signs of infection, perivascular administration of fluid, leakage of fluid from the catheter and giving set junction, or 'blowing' of the vein.
- Replace the sterile dressing daily.

Cleaning urinary catheters[9]

1. Flush, with force, copious amounts of cold water through the catheter immediately after use. This is usually done with a syringe. Cold water prevents coagulation of any protein that may be present.
2. Remove any blockages with a wire stylet and repeat step 1.
3. Wash the exterior and interior of the catheter with a mild detergent. Rinse thoroughly, as in step 1.
4. Check catheter for kinks, holes, etc. If any damage is found the catheter must be discarded.
5. Dry in a warm, dust-free atmosphere.

Selection of feeding tubes[2]

Feeding tube	Duration	Advantages	Disadvantages
Naso-oesophageal	Short term (<5 days)	Inexpensive. Easy to place. General anaesthesia not required	Requires liquid diet. Some animals will not eat voluntarily with tube in place
Oesophagostomy	Long term	Inexpensive. Easy to place. Can use energy-dense diets	Requires anaesthesia. Cellulitis is major complication seen
Gastrostomy	Long term	Can use energy-dense diets	Requires anaesthesia and/or surgery
Jejunostomy	Long term	Bypasses stomach and duodenum. Can be used in patients with pancreatitis	Requires anaesthesia and laparotomy. For in-hospital use. Requires continuous rate infusion. Requires liquid diet

Calculating resting energy requirement (RER)[1]

The following equation can be used to calculate the RER in kcal/day for cats or dogs:

$$RER = 70 \times \text{bodyweight (kg)}^{0.75}$$

Alternatively, for animals over 2 kg the following equation can be used:

$$RER = 30 \times \text{bodyweight (kg)} + 70$$

Note: To convert kcal to kilojoules (kJ) multiply by 4.185

Nursing considerations for feeding tubes[2]

Managing patients with feeding tubes requires special attention. Oesophagostomy, gastrostomy and jejunostomy tubes are secured in place with sutures and the tubes are then bandaged. The dressings and bandages should be inspected daily for any sign of infection and the site cleaned. After each use, all feeding tubes should be flushed with water to prevent clogging. Prevention of premature removal of tubes can be accomplished by using Elizabethan collars and by bandaging tubes securely. Care should be taken to avoid wrapping too tightly as this could lead to patient discomfort and even compromise proper ventilation.

As enteral diets are mostly composed of water (most canned food are already >75% water) the amount of fluids administered parenterally should be adjusted accordingly to avoid volume overload.

The majority of complications from feeding tubes involve tube occlusion or localized irritation at the tube exit site. More serious complications include infection at the exit site or, rarely, complete tube dislodgment and peritonitis (gastrostomy or jejunostomy tube). Complications can be avoided by using the appropriate tube, effectively securing the tube, proper diet selection and preparation and careful monitoring.

Physiotherapy[6]

Positional physiotherapy

1. Encourage the patient to stand at regular intervals.
2. Support the patient in sternal recumbency with sandbags, cushions or rolled-up towels.
3. Maintain each position for 10–15 minutes, three or four times daily.
4. Between treatment sessions, turn laterally recumbent patient on a regular basis every 2–4 hours throughout the day and night.

Local hypothermia

5–10 minutes every 4–6 hours

Physiological effects	Results
↓ Tissue temperature, vasoconstriction, ↓ nerve conduction, relaxation of skeletal muscle	Analgesia, ↓ oedema, ↓ bruising

Superficial hyperthermia

10–20 minutes, 4–6 times a day

Physiological effects	Results
↑ Tissue temperature, vasodilation, ↑ local circulation, ↑ metabolic rate	Relief of muscle tension, analgesia, ↓ oedema

Massage

10–20 minutes, 2–3 times per day

Physiological effects	Results
Assisted venous return to the heart, ↑ lymphatic flow, ↑ muscular motion, ↑ tissue perfusion, maintained and improved peripheral circulation	↓ Oedema, ↓ muscle tension and spasm, temporary analgesia, ↑ muscle tone, ↑ movement through stretching of adhesions, ↓ heart rate

Passive exercise

10–20 minutes, 2–3 times a day following massage

Physiological effects	Results
Stretched adhesions, maintained or improved blood and lymphatic flow, stimulated sensory nerves	Prevention or ↑ range of movement, prevention or improvement of contractures, improved microcirculation to muscles and joints, improvement of stiffness

➡

1. The patient should be comfortable, supported in lateral recumbency with the affected limb uppermost. Sandbags can be used to give additional support.
2. Use one hand to stabilize the limb above or below the joint during manipulation.
3. Use the other hand for manipulation of the joint.
4. Manipulate the distal joints of the limb first, i.e. put each toe through its full range of movement.
5. Then, working up the limb, put each joint through its full range of movement as far as the hip or shoulder.
6. Move the whole limb passively in a normal ambulatory fashion.
7. When the movement at a joint is restricted, gentle overpressure can be used at the end of the range of movement.
8. As treatment progresses, range of movement at the restricted joint improves slowly.

The aim is to move each joint individually through its full range. In recumbent patients the uppermost limbs are manipulated first. The patient can then be turned and the process repeated on other limbs.

Active movement

Treatment sessions last from a few seconds, proceeding up to 10 minutes as the patient gains strength

Physiological effects	Results
↑ Blood supply and lymphatic drainage, ↑ muscular tone	Gradual build-up of muscular tone and strength, improved balance and coordination, patient comfort and stimulation

Stages of active exercise and movement

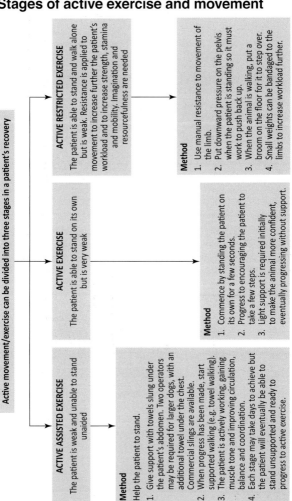

Active movement/exercise can be divided into three stages in a patient's recovery

ACTIVE ASSISTED EXERCISE

The patient is weak and unable to stand unaided

Method

Help the patient to stand.

1. Give support with towels slung under the patient's abdomen. Two operators may be required for larger dogs, with an additional towel under the chest. Commercial slings are available.
2. When progress has been made, start supported walking (e.g. towel walking).
3. The patient is actively working, gaining muscle tone and improving circulation, balance and coordination.
4. Each stage may take days to achieve but the patient will eventually be able to stand unsupported and ready to progress to active exercise.

ACTIVE EXERCISE

The patient is able to stand on its own but is very weak

Method

1. Commence by standing the patient on its own for a few seconds.
2. Progress to encouraging the patient to take a few steps.
3. Light support is required initially to make the animal more confident, eventually progressing without support.

ACTIVE RESTRICTED EXERCISE

The patient is able to stand and walk alone but is weak. Resistance is applied to increase further the patient's workload and to increase strength, stamina and mobility. Imagination and resourcefulness are needed

Method

1. Use manual resistance to movement of the limb.
2. Put downward pressure on the pelvis when the patient is standing so it must work to push back up.
3. When the animal is walking, put a broom on the floor for it to step over.
4. Small weights can be bandaged to the limbs to increase workload further.

NOTES

NOTES

NOTES

PART 3

Laboratory

Blood

Arterial blood sampling[1]

Indications/Use

- To obtain a sample of arterial blood for assessment of respiratory function or acid–base status

Contraindications

- Coagulopathy
- Sampling should not be performed at sites where risk of bacterial contamination and infection are high, e.g. due to local tissue damage, local skin infection, diarrhoea, urinary incontinence

Equipment

- Hypodermic needle:
  - Cats: 23–25 G; $5/8$ inch
  - Dogs: 23 G; $5/8$ inch
- 2 ml syringe
- Heparin sodium: this is used to pre-coat the syringe and needle used for blood collection; approximately 0.5 ml of heparin sodium is aspirated into the 2 ml syringe via the needle and then expelled. Alternatively, pre-heparinized blood-gas syringes with needles attached can be used
- 70% surgical spirit
- Cotton wool or gauze swabs
- 25 mm wide adhesive tape

Patient preparation and positioning

- Arterial blood sampling is performed in the conscious animal.
- Sedation should be avoided if possible as it will affect the result of blood gas analysis.
- Animals should be positioned appropriately for the blood collection site (see below).

Sites: Most commonly the dorsal pedal artery is used, but in cats and small dogs it is sometimes easier to use the femoral artery.

Dorsal pedal artery
- The animal is placed in lateral recumbency, either on a table (cats and small dogs) or on the floor (large dogs), with the leg to be sampled placed closest to the table or floor.
- An assistant restrains the patient's head with one hand and the uppermost hindlimb with the other.
- The artery is palpated just distal to the tarsus (hock), between the second and third metatarsal bones.

Femoral artery
- The animal is placed in lateral recumbency, either on a table (cats and small dogs) or on the floor (large dogs), with the leg to be sampled placed closest to the table or floor.
- The animal is restrained manually, and the upper limb abducted so that the femoral artery can be palpated.
- The femoral artery pulse is palpable on the medial thigh, ventral to the inguinal region and proximal to the stifle.

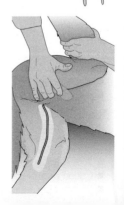

Technique

1. Stretch the skin over the artery.
2. Palpate the artery so that its pulsation can be felt.
3. The skin overlying the artery is clipped, then sprayed or lightly wiped with surgical spirit. Excessive scrubbing/wiping of the skin should be avoided, as this may result in spasm of the artery.
4. Direct the needle, with syringe attached, toward the palpated artery, at an angle of about 30 degrees. The needle bevel is pointed upwards.
5. Penetrate the artery in one quick firm purposeful movement.
6. When the artery has been penetrated, a flash of blood will be seen in the hub of the needle.
7. Collect approximately 1 ml of blood.
8. Remove the syringe and needle from the artery.
9. On removal of the needle, apply direct pressure to the artery for 5 minutes, then cover with cotton wool or a gauze swab and adhesive tape.
10. Hold the syringe upright and tap it to cause air bubbles to rise. Eject any air from the syringe.
11. Cap the sample with an airtight seal to prevent exposure to room air. Rubber bungs or plastic caps are available with pre-heparinized blood-gas syringes.
12. The blood sample must be analysed within 5 minutes.

Potential complications

- Significant haemorrhage is very uncommon, provided direct pressure is applied to the artery (see above)
- Bruising and the formation of a small haematoma will occur in some patients, but can be minimized by good technique and by the application of direct pressure to the artery
- Arterial thrombosis is uncommon but is more likely if repeated attempts are made to collect blood from an artery

Venous blood sampling[1]

Indications/Use
- To obtain a sample of venous blood for clinical pathology tests or for bacterial culture

Contraindications
- Coagulopathy
- Sampling should not be performed at sites where risk of bacterial contamination and infection are high, e.g. due to local tissue damage, local skin infection, diarrhoea, urinary incontinence

Equipment
- Hypodermic needles:
    - Cats: 23–21 G; $5/8$ inch
    - Dogs: 21 G; $5/8$ inch or 1 inch
- 2–10 ml syringes
- 70% surgical spirit
- 4% chlorhexidine gluconate or 10% povidone–iodine
- Cotton wool or gauze swabs
- 25 mm wide adhesive tape
- Appropriate blood containers (see table below) and/or three blood culture bottles (pre-warmed to 37°C)
- Sterile gloves

EDTA (ethylene diamine tetra-acetic acid)	
Universal *	Pink/red
Vacutainer *	Lavender or pink
Sample	Whole blood
Tests	Haematology
Comments	Fill tube precisely to level indicated. Underfilling may cause artefacts; overfilling may lead to clotting

None	
Universal *	White/clear
Vacutainer *	Red
Sample	Serum
Tests	Biochemistry; bile acids; serology

Serum gel	
Universal *	Brown
Vacutainer *	Gold
Sample	Serum
Tests	Biochemistry; bile acids; serology

Lithium heparin	
Universal *	Orange or green
Vacutainer *	Green or green/orange
Sample	Plasma
Tests	Biochemistry; electrolytes
Comments	Do not use blood that has been mixed with EDTA

Sodium fluoride and potassium oxalate	
Universal *	Yellow
Vacutainer *	Grey
Sample	Whole blood
Tests	Blood glucose
Comments	Fluoride/oxalate inhibits red blood cells oxidizing glucose

Sodium citrate	
Universal *	Lilac
Vacutainer *	Light blue
Sample	Whole blood
Tests	Coagulation tests; platelet counts

*Always check cap colour codes, as manufacturers may vary ➡

Patient preparation and positioning

- Venous blood sampling is performed in the conscious animal, although in fractious animals light sedation may be required.
- The animal should be positioned appropriately for the blood collection site (see below).
- Clip the hair over the appropriate vein.
- Using cotton wool or gauze swabs, clean the skin over the vein with 4% chlorhexidine or 10% povidone–iodine, followed by spraying with surgical spirit.
- When taking samples for bacterial culture, take care not to touch the site of needle insertion. If necessary, gloves should be worn.

Sites: The jugular vein is preferred to peripheral veins in order to minimize the potential for cell damage during blood sampling. The cephalic vein and the lateral saphenous vein (which runs over the lateral aspect of the hock) may sometimes be used.

Jugular vein

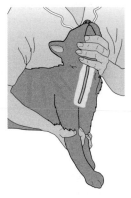

- The animal is placed in a sitting position, either on a table (cats and small dogs) or on the floor (large dogs).
- An assistant stands on the left of the patient.
- The assistant places their right arm over the patient's back and round the front of the patient, to encircle and control the forelimbs.
- The assistant's left arm is used to extend the animal's neck by grasping its muzzle and directing the nostrils towards the ceiling.

Cephalic vein

■ The animal is placed in a sitting position or in sternal recumbency, either on a table (cats and small dogs) or on the floor (large dogs).

■ An assistant stands on the left of the patient.

■ The assistant passes their left hand under the patient's neck and holds the head turned away from the sampler.

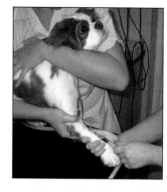

■ The assistant's right arm is used to extend the patient's right forelimb.

Saphenous vein

■ The animal is placed in lateral recumbency, either on a table (cats and small dogs) or on the floor (large dogs).

■ An assistant restrains the animal's head with one hand.

■ With the other hand, the assistant extends the uppermost hindlimb, at the same time stretching out the body. The hand is placed around the leg at the level of the mid-tibia/fibula.

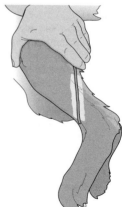

Technique

For biochemical tests or haematology:

1. Raise the vein by compressing it at a point closer to the heart than the venepuncture site.

2. Insert the needle, with syringe attached, into the vein with the bevel upwards, at an angle of approximately 30 degrees.

➤

3. Aspirate blood by withdrawing the syringe plunger. Avoid excessive suction on the syringe as this may collapse the vein.
4. Release the pressure on the vein.
5. Remove the needle and apply gentle pressure to the venepuncture site for a few seconds.
6. If the cephalic or saphenous veins are used, apply a light bandage of cotton wool held by adhesive tape for 30–60 minutes.
7. Place the blood sample in the appropriate tube(s).
8. Gently invert the sample tube several times to ensure adequate distribution of any additive. Do NOT shake the tube, as this may cause haemolysis.

For bacterial culture:

1. Follow steps 1 to 5 above to take a 5–10 ml blood sample (see culture bottle for required volume). Sterile examination gloves should be worn.

6. Place a new needle on the syringe.
7. Swab the rubber stopper of the culture bottle with surgical spirit and allow to dry.
8. Add the required volume of blood to the pre-warmed culture bottle.
9. Collect three blood samples with a minimum of 1 hour between samples OR, in acutely septic patients, all three samples can be taken over 30 minutes.
10. The culture bottles should be transported to the laboratory as quickly as possible. Although not ideal, overnight postage may still allow meaningful results.

Potential complications

These are very uncommon but may include:
- Minor haemorrhage
- Subcutaneous haematoma formation
- Vascular trauma
- Thrombophlebitis.

Changes in serum or plasma samples[9]

Colour	Reason for change
Pink/red	Haemolysed sample – red blood cells have been damaged due to incorrect sampling or preservation
Yellow	Icteric sample – the colour change is caused by the presence of bilirubin, which indicates liver damage
Milky white	Lipaemic sample – due to the presence of fat in unstarved animals or evidence of liver disease

PCV determination using a Hawksley reader[9]

1. Place the tube into the slot in the reader, with the sealed end downwards.
2. Align the top of the seal, i.e. the bottom of the red blood cell layer, with the zero line on the reader.

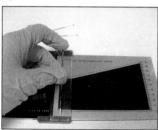

3. Move the tube holder across until the top of the plasma is lined up with the 100% line on the reader.

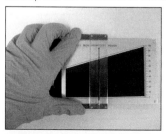

4. Move the adjustable PCV reading line to intersect the top of the RBC layer.

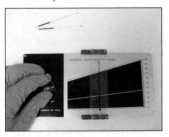

5. Record the PCV reading correctly as a percentage.

Preparation of a blood smear[1]

Indications/Use

■ Assessment of:
- Leucocyte (WBC) differential count
- Leucocyte abnormalities, e.g. toxic neutrophils, left shift, blast cells
- Red blood cell morphology, e.g. polychromasia, anisocytosis, fragmented red cells, spherocytes, Heinz bodies, red cell parasites
- Platelet count
- Platelet abnormalities, e.g. macroplatelets and platelet clumps

Equipment

■ Blood collected in an EDTA anticoagulant tube (see **Venous blood sampling** – page 34)
■ Microhaematocrit tube
■ Microscope slides
■ A 'spreader' slide: this is narrower than the smear slide to avoid spreading the cells over the edge of the slide. 'Spreaders' can be made by breaking the corner off a normal slide, having first scored it with a blade or diamond writer

Technique

1. Using a microhaematocrit tube, place a small drop of well mixed blood in the centre line toward one end of a microscope slide.

2. Hold the 'spreader' between the thumb and middle finger, placing the index finger on top of the 'spreader'.

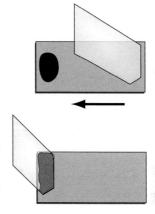

3. Place the 'spreader' in front of the blood spot, at an angle of about 30 degrees, and draw it backwards until it comes into contact with the blood, allowing the blood to spread out rapidly along the edge of the 'spreader'.

4. The moment this occurs, advance the 'spreader' forwards smoothly and quickly.

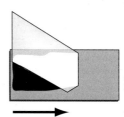

5. As the smear is made, a 'feathered edge' forms. *Do not lift the 'spreader' slide until the feathered edge is complete.*

6. Ideally the smear should extend approximately two-thirds of the length of the slide.

7. Allow the smear to air dry fully before staining with an appropriate stain.

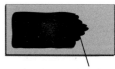

Feathered edge

Practical tips: common faults and how to avoid them

Fault	How to avoid
Film too thick	Use a smaller drop of blood
Film too thin	Use a larger drop of blood and/or faster spreading motion
Alternating thick and thin bands	Ensure spreading motion is smooth and avoid hesitation
Streaks along length of smear	Ensure edge of spreader is not irregular or coated with dried blood Ensure no dust on slide or in blood
'Holes' in smear	Ensure slide is free of grease
Narrow, thick smear	Allow blood to spread right across spreader slide before making smear

Staining procedures[9]

Leishman's
1. Put on gloves.
2. Place slide on staining rack with smear uppermost.
3. Cover with Leishman's stain and leave for 2 minutes.
4. Add twice the stain's volume of buffered distilled water pH 6.8 and gently mix using a Pasteur pipette.
5. Leave for 10–15 minutes.
6. Wash the slide with buffered distilled water pH 6.8.
7. Allow slide to dry.

Giemsa
1. Put on gloves.
2. Fix the slide by dipping in methanol for 1 minute.
3. Flood the slide with diluted Giemsa stain and leave for 30 minutes.
4. Rinse the slide with distilled water.
5. Allow slide to dry.

Diff-Quik

1. Put on gloves.
2. Dip slide into the fixative (methanol) solution (pale blue) five times. Allow excess fluid to drip back into the jar.
3. Dip slide into stain (eosin) solution 1 (red) five times. Allow excess fluid to drip back into the jar.
4. Dip slide into stain (methylene blue) solution 2 (purple) five times. Allow excess fluid to drip back into the jar.
5. Rinse slide with distilled water.
6. Place slide vertically and leave to dry.

Reference ranges for haematology values[9]

Species	RBC count (10^{12}/l)	WBC count (10^9/l)	PCV (%)	Hb (g/dl)	MCV (fl)	MCHC (g/dl)
Dog	5.5–8.5	6–17	37–55	12—18	60–70	32—36
Cat	5–10	5.5–19.5	24–45	9—17	39–55	30—36

Reference ranges for biochemistry values[9]

Biochemical parameter	Dogs	Cats
Albumin (g/l)	25–40	25–40
Alanine aminotransferase (ALT) (IU/l)	10–75	35–134
Alkaline phosphatase (ALP) (IU/l)	0–80	15–96
Blood urea nitrogen (mmol/l)	2.5–7	5–11
Calcium (mmol/l)	2–3	1.8–3
Cholesterol (mmol/l)	2.5–8	2–6.5
Creatinine (µmol/l)	40–130	40–130
Glucose (mmol/l)	3.3–6	3.3–6
Pancreatic amylase (IU/l)	350–1200	515–2210
Phosphate (mmol/l)	0.8–1.6	1.3–2.6
Total bilirubin (µmol/l)	1.7–10	2–5
Total protein (g/l)	54–71	54–78

NB Reference ranges will vary with laboratory; these are averages

Urine

Summary of urinalysis tests[6]

VISUAL INSPECTION

Assess colour and turbidity (cloudiness)

SPECIFIC GRAVITY (SG)

1. To calibrate refractometer, place distilled water beneath plastic cover of refractometer.
2. Adjust until SG = 1.000 and then dry refractometer.
3. Place urine under plastic cover of refractometer.
4. Read SG (the point where red area turns to white; in the example (right) the SG is 1.024).
5. Rinse and dry refractometer.

Note: Dipstick assessment of SG is inaccurate

DIPSTICK ANALYSIS (pH, glucose, ketones, protein, bilirubin)

1. Invert urine sample to ensure thorough mixing.
2. Cover all squares on dipstick with urine and note time.
3. Read dipstick results at times indicated on barrel.

Note: Dipstick SG is inaccurate and dipsticks will not detect all types of ketones

MICROSCOPIC EXAMINATION OF SEDIMENT

Examine as soon as possible after collection

1. Centrifuge 10 ml at 2000 rpm for 5 minutes.
2. Remove supernatant and re-suspend sediment by tapping tube.

Wet preparation:
■ Place a drop of suspension on a slide and stain with new methylene blue if necessary
■ Place a cover slip over the urine

Dry preparation:
■ Make a smear using a drop of re-suspended sediment
■ Rapidly air-dry and stain with Leishman's stain

Urine specific gravity (USG) normal values[6]

■ Dog   1.015–1.040
■ Cat   1.015–1.050
■ Rabbit   1.003–1.036

There can be variation from these ranges, depending on the age, breed, sex and hydration status of the animal.

Common faecal examinations [6]

Indications	Method
Gross examination	
Preliminary assessment	Assess: ■ Consistency and colour ■ Presence of mucus or fat ■ Presence of specific material (worms, foreign material, undigested food)
Direct smear	
Parasitic burden Undigested starch or muscle fibres	1. Place one drop of saline and one drop of faeces on slide. 2. Mix thoroughly; remove any large pieces of faecal material. 3. Smear and heat-fix, or cover with a cover slip. 4. Stain by placing a drop of stain at corner of cover slip and allow to spread. 5. Use 2% Lugol's iodine for starch (blue–black). 6. Use eosin, new methylene blue, Wright's for undigested muscle fibres. 7. Look for worm eggs under low power and Protozoa under medium power.
Faecal flotation	
Worm eggs Protozoa	1. Mix faeces with saturated sugar or zinc sulphate ($ZnSO_4$) solution [a]. (*Note:* Zinc sulphate flotation must be used for *Giardia* as other suspensions will cause destruction of this organism). 2. Ova and cysts will rise to surface, but centrifugation will improve sensitivity. 3. Examine supernatant within 15 minutes if looking for *Giardia*.
Faecal fat	
Undigested fat	1. Mix one drop of fresh faeces with one drop of Sudan III on a glass slide. 2. Examine microscopically. 3. Undigested fat will be seen as orange droplets.

[a] $ZnSO_4$ solution is made by mixing 331g of $ZnSO_4$ in 1 litre of water.

Hair and skin sampling procedures[6]

Hand-held lens examination

Indications
- Fleas, flea dirt, lice, and *Cheyletiella*

Equipment
- Low-power hand-held magnifying lens

Technique
Examine skin and hair with lens.

Wood's lamp

Indications
- Some strains of *Microsporum canis* fluoresce when exposed to ultraviolet light

Equipment
- Wood's lamp (ideally double tube); gloves; protective clothing; dark room

Technique
Allow lamp to warm up (5–10 minutes). In a dark room, expose hairs for 3–5 minutes (some are slow to respond). 50% of *Microsporum canis* will fluoresce apple green in colour. If positive, perform hair plucking and culture on dermatophyte test medium or Sabouraud's medium, or send to outside laboratory. *Note:* Some bacteria, skin debris or certain drugs may fluoresce and give false positive results.

Coat brushing

Indications
- Fleas, lice, *Cheyletiella*, dermatophytes (ringworm)

Equipment
- Fine-toothed comb; paper for collection of material; microscope slides; liquid paraffin; pipette; cover slips; microscope

Technique
Stand the patient over paper. Groom animal's coat with comb. Examine debris with hand-held magnifying lens. Place some debris on a slide with a drop of liquid paraffin and apply a cover slip. Examine under low power microscope. Use damp cotton wool to examine suspected flea dirt (turns reddish brown at edge of dirt). Samples for an outside laboratory should go into paper packs, e.g. Dermpacks.

Mackenzie brush

Indications
- Dermatophytes or spores of dermatophytes

Equipment
- Mackenzie brush; growth medium

Technique
Sterile toothbrush is brushed through coat to collect hairs. Press toothbrush on to dermatophyte test medium or Sabouraud's medium for culture.

Skin scraping

Indications
- For detection of all mites, particularly those living deep in the skin

Equipment
- Scissors or clippers; liquid paraffin; pipette; scalpel blade (size 10 or 15); microscope slides; cover slips; microscope

➡

Technique

Sedate the patient under veterinary direction if required (e.g. for scrapes from face, feet or painful lesions). Select areas of lesional skin (erythema, papules, scaling, alopecia). Clip hair *carefully* with scissors or clippers, taking care *not* to touch the skin surface. Pipette a drop of liquid paraffin on to skin or scalpel blade. Gently pinch up skin at selected site to help extrude mites/bacteria. Hold skin flat and taut and scrape with the scalpel blade at angle of 90 degrees to the skin until capillary ooze is seen. *Always scrape several sites.* Transfer scraping on to microscope slide(s). If the material on the slide is too thick it will be difficult to see anything. Divide material between slides. Add a small amount of liquid paraffin and apply cover slip. Clean scrape sites with dilute antiseptic. Examine slide(s) first under low power (x4) magnification to increase scanning speed. Use with condenser low, and light beam diaphragm half-closed to closed to optimize contrast. Increase magnification to x10 and systematically examine slide.

Note: Some types of mite are found in small numbers in normal animals. Some mites require collection of deep skin scrapes, whilst others can be detected on superficial skin scrapes.

Potassium hydroxide is sometimes used as it decolorizes skin and hair; however, it is caustic and kills the mites, making them hard to see.

Hair plucking

Indications
- Samples for fungal culture or trichograms, dermatophytes (ringworm), occasionally *Demodex*

Equipment
- Broad-rimmed epilation forceps; slides; liquid paraffin; gloves

Technique

Look for hairs immersed in scale and crust. Pluck single, entire hairs from the edges of lesions, using epilation.

For in-house examination: Place hair on slide. Add liquid paraffin or stain (lactophenol cotton blue or Quink black/blue ink). Examine under microscope. Affected material including hair shaft will stain blue.

For an outside laboratory: Place hair sample in clearly labelled paper envelope.

Sticky tape preparation – 1

Indications
■ Lice and *Cheyletiella*

Equipment
■ Scissors or clippers; clear sticky tape (19 mm wide); liquid paraffin; microscope slides; microscope

Technique

Select areas of dry scaly skin and scurfy hair. Clip hair carefully, avoiding skin surface. Apply sticky surface of adhesive tape to skin and base of hairs. Add a small drop of liquid paraffin to a microscope slide. Place tape (sticky side down) on to microscope slide. Examine immediately using low power objective.

Sticky tape preparation – 2

Indications
■ *Malassezia* and bacteria

Equipment
■ As above plus: Scotch tape 19 mm – other tapes unsuitable for staining
■ Diff-Quik or Rapi-Diff stains; tissues; microscope; immersion oil

Technique

Select area of greasy, erythematous skin (axillae, inguinal and interdigital regions). Clip hair *carefully*. Apply sticky surface of adhesive tape several times to skin. Stain sticky tape with Diff-Quik. Attach tape, sticky side down, to microscope slide. ➡

Cover with paper tissues and exert gentle pressure to remove excess fluid. Examine immediately using x40 or x100 under oil immersion.

Impression smears

Indications
- Cytological assessment or *Demodex*

Equipment
- Microscope slide; microscope

Technique
Slide is pressed directly against lesion and smeared. Air-dry slide. Stain for cytology. Examine under microscope

Fine needle aspiration

Indications
- *Demodex*, bacteria, cytology

Equipment
- Sterile 5 ml syringe; sterile 25 G needle; microscope slides; cover slip; microscope

Technique
Aspirate pustule or nodule contents using a sterile syringe and needle (see page 51). Express contents on to slide. Smear or place cover slip on top. Examine under microscope.

Skin biopsy

Indications
- Histopathology, dermatophytes, *Malassezia*, bacteria and occasionally mites

Equipment
- Biopsy punch or scalpel blade and handle; sterile swabs; 10% formalin in wide-mouthed container; shiny card; sterile needle; suture material and instruments

Technique

Clip hair carefully, avoiding skin. Collect sample, using biopsy punch or an elliptical incision. Blot off excess fluid with a sterile swab (so that it does not slip off the card). Using a sterile needle, place dermal layer in contact with shiny card. Place in 10% formalin immediately (cells deteriorate very quickly if left exposed to air). Close skin with a single suture.

Fine needle aspiration of a mass[6]

1. Lay out at least five slides on a clean surface and draw back an empty 10 ml syringe.
2. Clip the area to be aspirated and clean with spirit.
3. Immobilize the mass if possible (aspirates of body organs should be performed with ultrasound guidance).

Needle-only technique:

1. Insert the needle into the mass and move it rapidly in and out (to ensure cells are broken away from the tissue).
2. Remove the needle and attach to a syringe containing 10 ml of air.

Fine needle aspiration with suction:

1. With the needle attached to the syringe, insert the needle into the mass.
2. Draw back on the syringe to the 5 ml mark (this should be quite difficult because of negative pressure created).
3. Whilst maintaining suction, move the needle around within the mass.
4. Release suction before removing the needle from the mass.
5. Remove needle from end of syringe, draw 10 ml air into the syringe and reattach to the needle.

Making the smear:

1. With the bevel of the needle facing down, squirt out the contents of the needle on to one end of a clean slide.
2. Make a smear or a squash preparation.

Squash preparation[1]

1. Expel the aspirate on to the centre of a microscope slide.

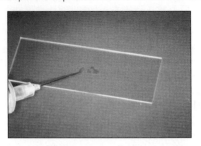

2. Place a second 'spreader' slide horizontally and at right angles to spread the sample, taking care not to exert too much downward pressure to avoid rupturing the cells.

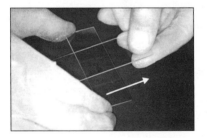

3. Draw the 'spreader' slide quickly and smoothly across the bottom slide. **Note that it is the smear produced on the *underside of the 'spreader' slide* that is examined with the microscope.**

Packaging laboratory samples for external analysis[6]

Labelling and paperwork

Each sample should be labelled with the owner's name, the animal's name or reference number, the type of sample collected and the date of collection (e.g. 'Fluffy Brown – Urine 24/2/12').

An appropriate submission form should accompany every sample submitted to an external laboratory. If a submission form is not available, similar information should be provided in an accompanying letter. This information ensures that the laboratory performs the appropriate test and is able to interpret the results. Forms should be placed in a plastic envelope to prevent contamination should the container break in transit.

Information required by external laboratories
■ Name and address of submitting veterinary surgeon
■ Owner's name
■ Animal's name or reference number
■ Species, breed, age and sex (M, MN, F, FN)
■ Date of sampling and time of collection
■ Clinical history, including presenting signs, and current treatments
■ Types of samples collected (including type of preservatives used)
■ Site(s) of sample collection
■ Test or examination required

Postage and packaging

Samples that are not preserved, packed or posted appropriately may be damaged in transit. Damaged samples can produce inaccurate results and it is therefore extremely important to ensure that samples arrive in the best possible condition.

- Check the information supplied by the laboratory to ensure that the correct types of sample are being sent.
- Do not post samples on a Friday, as they will sit in a warm post box all weekend.

➡

The following are rules for postage of pathological samples, and
must be adhered to.

- The sender must ensure that the sample will not expose
  anyone to danger (COSHH 1988).
- A *maximum* sample of *50 ml* is allowed through the post,
  unless by specific arrangement with Royal Mail.
- Samples must be labelled correctly with time, date, owner
  and animal identification, and nature of the sample
  (e.g. 'heparinized plasma').
- *Primary container* must be leak-proof and must be wrapped
  in enough absorbent material to absorb the complete
  sample if leakage or breakage occurs.
- The wrapped sample is then placed in a *leak-proof
  plastic bag*.
- This is placed in a *secondary container* (e.g. polypropylene
  clip-down container or cylindrical metal container).
- Seal the correctly completed *laboratory form* in a plastic
  bag for extra protection and place with sample.
- Place in a *tertiary container* (strong cardboard or grooved
  polystyrene box), approved by Royal Mail, and seal
  securely.
- *Outer packaging must be labelled conspicuously:*
  'FRAGILE WITH CARE / PATHOLOGICAL SPECIMEN /
  ADDRESS OF LABORATORY / Address of sender.
- Send by *first-class letter post* (*not* parcel post).

WARNING
If the Royal Mail's conditions are not complied with
the sender is liable to prosecution.

NOTES

NOTES

PART 4

Bandaging and wound care

Wound dressings[6]

Dry

Dry-to-dry

- **Description:** Sterile gauze swabs
- **Characteristics:** Dry swabs placed on wound to absorb exudates. Adheres to necrotic tissue
- **Indications:**
  - Exuding wounds
  - Necrotic wounds
  - Not recommended on granulating wounds

Wet-to-dry

- **Description:** Sterile gauze swabs soaked in sterile saline
- **Characteristics:** Dry swabs soaked in sterile saline applied on wound. Adheres to necrotic tissue
- **Indications:**
  - Exuding wounds
  - Necrotic wounds
  - Not recommended on granulating wounds

Non-adherent – 1

- **Description:** Perforated polyester film, absorbent, 80% cotton, 20% viscose pad non-woven backing material
- **Characteristics:** Shiny side down on wound. Does not absorb exudates and can adhere to exuding wounds. Needs secondary dressings

- **Examples:** Rondopad (Millpledge), Melolin (Smith & Nephew), Primapore (Smith & Nephew)
- **Indications:**
    - Dry wounds
    - Postoperative wounds
    - Sutures

Non-adherent – 2

- **Description:** Bleached cotton/rayon cloth impregnated with white or yellow soft paraffin
- **Characteristics:** Paraffin reduces adherence to wound but can dry out if not changed regularly. Needs secondary dressing
- **Examples:** Jelonet (Smith & Nephew), Grassolind (Millpledge)
- **Indications:**
    - Clean superficial wounds
    - Abrasions
    - Cuts

Interactive

Hydrogels

- **Description:** 2.3% modified sodium carboxymethylcellulose polymer, 77.7% water, 20% propylene glycol, 3.5% starch grafted polymer aqueous base, 20% propylene glycol
- **Characteristics:** Available as flat sheets or gels. Have high water content; can rehydrate wounds and ensure moist wound healing. Cool surface of wound. Too much can cause maceration. Can be mixed with topical medications. Need secondary dressing
- **Examples:** IntraSite (Smith & Nephew), Aquaform
- **Indications:**
    - Desloughing
    - Exuding wounds
    - Abscess cavities

Hydrocolloids

- ***Description:*** Microgranular suspension of polymers – consists of a waterproof polyurethane foam bonded on a polyurethane film that acts as carrier for hydrocolloid base
- ***Characteristics:*** Absorbs exudates into foam, leading to change in the dressing. Should be 2 cm or more either side of the wound edges. Does not require a secondary dressing
- ***Examples:*** Granuflex (ConvaTec), Tegasorb (3M)
- ***Indications:*** Light to medium exuding wounds

Foam

- ***Description:*** Absorbent polyurethane containing either hydrocellular or hydropolymer foam and some carbon. Comes in a variety of forms
- ***Characteristics:*** Can absorb 6–10 times own weight in exudates. Conforms to cavity. White surface placed on wound. Exudate does not leak through. Works by capillary action drawing exudates from wound. Needs secondary dressings. Can be left in place for up to 7 days
- ***Examples:*** Allevyn (Smith & Nephew), Lyofoam (Acme United)
- ***Indications:***
    - Suitable for all types of wounds that have light to heavy exudates
    - Deep cavity wounds

Alginate

- ***Description:*** Made from a variety of seaweeds, some contain calcium. Mixed into a non-woven dressing
- ***Characteristics:*** Highly absorbent; dressings turn to gel once mixed with exudates. Some have haemostatic properties. Needs secondary dressings. Can be left in place for up to 7 days
- ***Examples:*** Algisite (Smith & Nephew), Kaltostat (ConvaTec)
- ***Indications:***
    - Infected wounds
    - Exuding wounds
    - Cavities
    - Haemorrhage

➥

Collagen

- ***Description:*** Collagen matrix
- ***Characteristics:*** Binds blood clotting factors XII and XIII. Causes natural wound cleansing. Attracts granulocytes and fibroblasts to the wound and forms an organized structure for basal cells of epidermis
- ***Examples:*** Vet BioSISt (Arnolds), Emovet (Nelson), Collamend (Genetrix)
- ***Indications:***
  - Most types of wounds
  - Not recommended for full thickness burns or necrotic wounds

Silver-coated dressings

- ***Description:*** SILCRYST; nanocrystals
- ***Characteristics:*** Silver ions released into wound bed. Have anti-inflammatory action and kills bacteria rapidly
- ***Examples:*** Acticoat (Smith & Nephew)
- ***Indications:*** Infected wounds

Vapour-permeable film

- ***Description:*** Thin conformable adhesive films
- ***Characteristics:*** Provides thin vapour-permeable film, allowing vapour exchange and maintenance of moist wound environment
- ***Examples:*** Opsite Flexigrid (Smith & Nephew), Tegaderm (3M)
- ***Indications:***
  - Uninfected shallow wounds
  - Intact skin at risk of pressure or maceration injury

Barrier film

- ***Description:*** Spray or foam containing polymer
- ***Characteristics:*** Sprayed over wound; dries to leave film of polymer that is permeable to moisture vapour and air. Creates a barrier
- ***Examples:*** Opsite (Smith & Nephew), Cavilon (3M), Film dressing spray (Millpledge)

- ■ *Indications:*
  - – Minor wounds
  - – Abrasions
  - – Sutures
  - – Wound covering on reptiles

Topical

Antiseptics

- ■ *Description:* Dilute chlorhexidine 0.05%; dilute povidone–iodine 1%
- ■ *Characteristics:* Used for initial cleansing of wounds. These solutions can be toxic to fibroblasts and should be avoided if possible. Contaminated wounds would be better treated with debridement
- ■ *Examples:* Hibitane, Pevidine, antiseptic solution
- ■ *Indications:* Contaminated wounds

Aloe vera

- ■ *Description:* Gel
- ■ *Characteristics:* Promotes wound healing by accelerating formation of granulation tissue. Stabilizes fibroblast growth factors and activates macrophages
- ■ *Examples:* Acemannan (Forever Living Products)
- ■ *Indications:* All wounds   ➡

NOTES

Hydrophilic cream

- **Description:** Hydrophilic cream containing silver sulfadiazine
- **Characteristics:** Inhibits growth of bacteria and fungi *in vitro*. Studies have been carried out to show antibacterial action against meticillin-resistant *Staphylococcus aureus*, *Pseudomonas* spp. and enterococci. Cream must be placed in wound as it will macerate surrounding skin
- **Examples:** Flamazine (Smith & Nephew)
- **Indications:** Burn wounds and wounds infected with Gram-negative bacteria

Sugar paste and honey

- **Description:** Paste. Caster sugar and additive-free icing sugar dissolved in hydrogen peroxide and polyethylene glycol 400 has been developed for clinical use
- **Characteristics:** Has been used in wounds for centuries. Paste has lower pH than wound and helps to debride infected or dirty wounds. Not suitable for granulating wounds. Honey must be sterile; has a high osmotic pressure and helps to draw out exudate
- **Indications:** Infected dirty wounds

Robert Jones bandage[6]

1. Place two lengths of zinc oxide tape to cover 15–20 cm up the leg and 10–13 cm overlap at the toes and place on each side of the leg to form stirrups. Pad out toes as necessary.
2. Place cotton wool layer: start halfway up nail and reverse roll cotton wool four or five times around the leg.

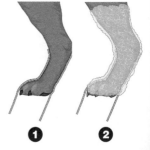

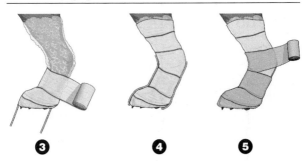

3. Place conforming bandage: this should compress the cotton wool as firmly and as evenly as possible and should cover it entirely.
4. Unstick two ends of zinc oxide tape and fold back to secure the bandage.
5. Cover the bandage with cohesive dressing.

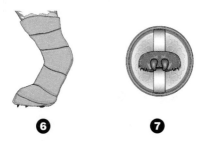

6. Check that the bandage is not too tight: it should be possible to insert two fingers between the bandage and the animal. When flicked, the bandage should sound like a ripe melon.
7. The two middle toes should remain exposed.

Ear and head bandage[6]

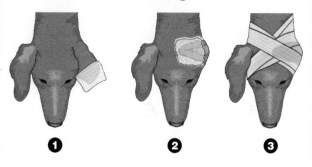

1. Cover any wounds with an appropriate sterile dressing.
2. Place padding on top of cranium. Pick up ear by tip of pinna and lay flat back on padding; repeat if including both ears. Place padding on top of pinna.
3. Place padding under neck. Wrap conforming layer in a figure-of-eight pattern until the area is covered, using the free ear for additional anchorage.

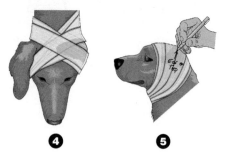

4. Cover the bandage with a cohesive layer following a similar pattern.
5. Use marker pen to indicate on the outer layer the position of the pinna. Make sure that the bandage does not interfere with swallowing or breathing.

Thoracic bandage[6]

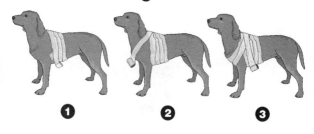

1. Apply a sterile dressing to any wound(s). Starting dorsally mid thorax apply a padding layer around the chest wall.
2. Incorporate the forelimbs in a figure-of-eight to help secure the bandage.
3. Return back along the chest wall, ending caudally to where the bandage started.

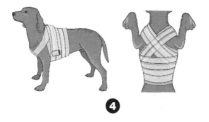

4. Cover the padded layer with a conforming bandage. Make sure that the bandage is not too tight and does not compromise respiratory efforts.

Abdominal bandage[6]

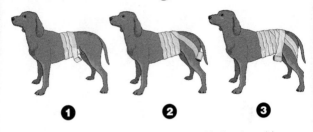

1. Apply a sterile dressing to any wound(s). Starting mid abdomen, apply a padding layer around the abdominal wall.
2. Incorporate the hindlimbs in a figure-of-eight to help secure the bandage.
3. Return back along the abdominal wall, ending cranially to where the bandage started.

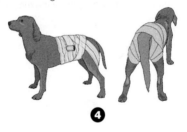

Cover the padded layer with a conforming bandage. Pay particular attention to anatomy of genitalia in both male and female – be careful not to cover prepuce or vulva.

Foot and lower limb bandage[6]

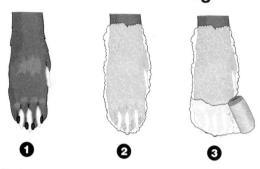

1. Cut long claws. Pad out the toes using a small piece of absorbent dressing.
2. Apply a padding layer over the foot covering the dorsal and palmar/plantar area.
3. Twist the bandage to cover diagonally the medial and lateral aspect of the foot.

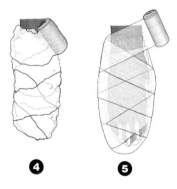

4. Roll the bandage in a proximal direction spiralling up the leg to cover the joint above the area to be bandaged.
5. Repeat this for the conforming layer and the cohesive layer.

Velpeau sling[6]

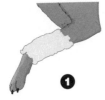 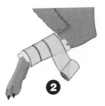

1. Pad the carpal area.
2. Secure conforming bandage over the carpal area, from lateral to medial.

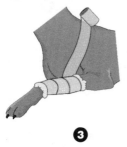 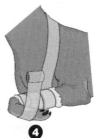

3. Bring the bandage from the medial carpus, up over the lateral aspect of the shoulder and around the opposite side of the chest behind the contralateral elbow.
4. Ensure the carpus, elbow and shoulder are flexed, and incorporate the carpus into the sling.
5. Repeat this until the complete forelimb has been covered, producing a sling effect. The whole bandage can be covered with a cohesive layer. Tension of the bandage must be checked carefully on application: if too tight it could result in ischaemic damage to the lower limb.

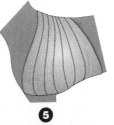

Ehmer sling[6]

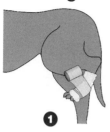 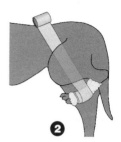

1. Lightly pad the metatarsal area (this prevents swelling, though too much padding will cause the bandage to slip). Secure conforming bandage around the metatarsal area from the medial to the lateral aspect.
2. Flex the whole limb, turning the foot inwards (this will turn the hock outwards and the stifle inwards, immobilizing the hip). Bring the bandage up under the medial aspect of the stifle. A small amount of padding may be applied to the cranial aspect of the stifle.

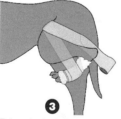 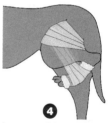

3. Bring the bandage over the lateral aspect of the thigh and around the medial aspect of the hock, returning to the lateral aspect of the metatarsals.
4. Apply several more layers until the leg is secure and the hip is supported. Repeat this for the cohesive dressing as required. Tension of the bandage must be checked carefully on application: if too tight, it could result in ischaemic damage to the lower limb.

Tail bandage[6]

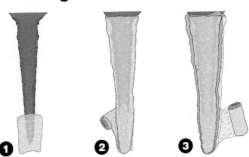

1. Use an appropriate dressing to cover the wound.
2. Using a conforming bandage, roll from the base, along the dorsal aspect of the tail, to the tip of the tail. Go under the tip, along the ventral aspect of the tail and back to the base.
3. Fold the bandage back on itself and return along the ventral surface to the tip of the tail.

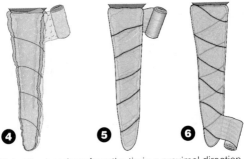

4. Spiral the bandage from the tip in a proximal direction towards the base, ensuring even pressure up to the base of the tail.
5. Apply a cohesive layer using the same methodology; from tip to base.
6. Return from base to tip.

Management of wound drains[6]

- Use aseptic techniques for all postoperative drain care.
- Clip a large area of hair around the wound, especially the area dependent to the wound.
- Use petroleum jelly or barrier spray to protect the skin dependent to the drain exit hole from maceration.
- Clean the exposed drain and skin exit holes twice daily with an antiseptic solution, such as povidone–iodine.
- Empty and change active suction devices as often as required to maintain function.
- Cover with a sterile dressing and light bandage. Change as often as necessary to prevent wound fluid penetrating to the outer dressing layer (strikethrough) and to maintain asepsis.
- Prevent patient interference with the drain.
- Drains are kept in place no longer than necessary, typically 2–5 days, until drainage has almost ceased. Some fluid will always be produced by a wound with a drain due to tissue reaction to the drain itself. The risks of complications increase with the time for which the drain is in place.

Complications of using drains include:

- Wound infection
- Wound dehiscence
- Early loss or removal from wound
- Failure of drainage
- Irritation and pain
- Drain tract cellulitis.

NOTES

NOTES

NOTES

NOTES

PART 5

Triage and emergency care

Fluid therapy

Clinical signs of dehydration[6]

Dehydration level	Clinical signs
<5%	Not detectable
5–6%	Subtle loss of skin elasticity
6–8%	Marked loss of skin elasticity Slightly prolonged capillary refill time Slightly sunken eyes Dry mucous membranes
10–12%	Tented skin stands in place Capillary refill time >2 seconds Sunken eyes Dry mucous membranes
12–15%	Early shock Moribund Death imminent

Calculating fluid loss using PCV[6]

If a 4.5 kg dehydrated cat has a PCV of 43%, how much fluid can it be estimated has been lost?

- Normal cat PCV = 35%
- Current PCV = 43%
- Increase = 8%
- For every 1% increase in PCV, animal requires 10 ml fluid/kg
- 8% increase in PCV = 8 x 10 ml x 4.5 kg = 360 ml

Answer : 360 ml of fluid

Calculating fluid loss using bodyweight[6]

Prior to illness, a Border Terrier weighed 12 kg. Following an episode of vomiting and diarrhoea, the same animal was found to weigh 11.2 kg. How much fluid can it be estimated to have lost?

- Difference in bodyweight = 12 kg – 11.2 kg = 0.8 kg (800 g)
- 1 kg = 1 litre, therefore 800 g = 800 ml

Answer : 800 ml

Estimating fluid loss due to known losses[6]

A 12 kg dog has vomited twice and had one episode of diarrhoea. Estimate the fluid loss.

- Vomit = 2 x 4 ml/kg x 12 kg = 96 ml
- Diarrhoea = 1 x 4 ml/kg x 12 kg = 48 ml
- Total = 144 ml

Answer : 144 ml

Calculating fluid rates[6]

Example 1

A 14 kg collie is found to be 10% dehydrated. The fluid is to be given over 8 hours. The giving set delivers 20 drops/ml. Calculate the drip rate to '1 drop every X seconds'.

1. Fluid lost = 10% of 14 kg dog = 10/100 x 14 kg = 1.4 kg
   1.4 kg = 1400 g = 1400 ml
2. Maintenance requirement = 50 ml/kg/day
   50 ml/kg x 14 kg = 700 ml
3. Fluid lost plus fluid maintenance = 1400 ml + 700 ml = 2100 ml
4. To be given over 8 hours, as stated:
   2100 ml ÷ 8 hours = 262.5 ml/hour
   262.5 ml/hour ÷ 60 minutes = 4.37 ml/minute
5. 4.37 ml/minute x giving set rate of 20 = 87.4 drops/minute
6. 60 ÷ 87.4 drops/minute = 0.68 (round up to 1)

Answer : 1 drop every 1 second.

NOTES

Crystalloid solutions[9]

Crystalloid solution	Ions (mmol/l)				Tonicity relative to extracellular fluid
	Na+	K+	Cl−	Ca2+	
Replacement					
Hartmann's solution	131	5	111	2	Isotonic
Lactated Ringer's solution	130	4	109	1.5	Isotonic
0.9% NaCl ('normal' saline)	154	0	154	0	Isotonic
Maintenance					
0.45% NaCl + 2.5% dextrose (glucose) (requires additional potassium)	77	0	77	0	Hypotonic
Normosol-M + 5% dextrose (glucose)	40	13	40	0	Mildly hypertonic
Others					
0.45% NaCl ('half strength' saline)	77	0	77	0	Hypotonic
0.9% NaCl + 5% glucose	154	0	154	0	Hypertonic
7.2% NaCl (hypertonic saline)	1232	0	1232	0	Hypertonic

Colloid solutions[6]

Colloid type	Example product names	Duration of action	Rate of fluid administration
Gelatins	Gelofusine	Up to 6 hours	Maximum dose: 20 ml/kg/24 hours
Starch (hetastarch, pentastarch)	elo-HAES, HAES-steril, Hemohes, Voluven, Volulyte	24–36 hours	Maximum dose: 20 ml/kg/24 hours

Blood transfusion

Calculating blood loss[6]

The volume of blood lost can be measured accurately using the following technique:

1. Calculate the weight of a dry swab.
2. Multiply this by the number of swabs used during the surgery (in order to calculate their dry weight).
3. Subtract this dry weight from the weight of the blood-soaked swabs to calculate the weight of the blood lost during the surgery.
4. Divide this weight by 1.3 to convert it into millilitres of blood (1 ml blood weighs 1.3 g).

> **Example:**
>
> 100 dry swabs weigh 230 g. Hence, one dry swab weighs 2.3 g (230/100).
>
> During an operation, the 20 blood-soaked swabs used are found to weigh 110 g. When dry, the 20 swabs would weigh 46 g (2.3 x 20). Therefore the blood must weigh 64 g (110 – 46). Hence the swabs contained 49 ml of blood (64/1.3).

Alternatively, a good estimate of the patient's blood loss can be calculated using the following technique:

1. Find out the volume of water needed to saturate 10 swabs.
2. Divide this by 10 for the volume of water needed to saturate one swab.
3. This is roughly equivalent to the volume of blood that will be contained in one swab.
4. Multiply the volume of blood contained in one saturated swab by the number of swabs used in the surgery to estimate the volume of blood lost.

> **Example:**
>
> If 10 swabs will absorb 50 ml of water, one swab will absorb 5 ml. During an operation, 14 swabs become saturated in blood. An estimate of the volume of blood soaked into these swabs is 70 ml (14 x 5).

When using either technique, remember to subtract the volume of any lavage fluids that have been used and that have also been soaked up by the swabs.

Collection [1,2]

Donor selection

In the UK, the collection of blood from healthy animals is governed by the RCVS and Home Office guidelines. Readers are advised to consult the relevant documents prior to blood collection.

Dogs

- Healthy, fully vaccinated, not receiving medication (except flea-preventive or routine worming medication)
- Suitable temperament
- >25 kg lean bodyweight
- 1–8 years of age
- Normal PCV, preferably >40%
- Ideally DEA 1.1-negative
- Nulliparous
- No history of a previous blood transfusion
- No history of travel outside the UK
- Blood can be collected every 4–6 weeks without the need for iron supplementation

Cats

- Healthy, fully vaccinated, not receiving medication (except flea-preventive or routine worming medication)
- Suitable temperament
- >4 kg lean bodyweight
- 1–8 years of age
- PCV >35%
- Blood typed (A, B or AB)
- No history of a previous blood transfusion
- No history of travel outside the UK
- Negative for FeLV, FIV, *Mycoplasma felis*
- Blood can be collected every 4–6 weeks without the need for iron supplementation

Owners of blood donors need to:

- Be available within a 10–15-minute drive from the practice to allow for speedy donation of blood in emergency situations
- Agree to try to bring their animal to the practice at short notice whenever possible
- Notify the practice if they are on holiday
- Contact the practice should their animal become unwell or be receiving medication so that it can temporarily be removed from the register
- Continue with regular vaccination of their animal.

Equipment

- As required for aseptic preparation
- Blood collection containers:
    - Dogs: standard commercial blood collection bag containing an anticoagulant, such as citrate phosphate dextrose (CPD), citrate phosphate dextrose adenine (CPDA) or acid citrate dextrose (ACD), attached to an extension tube and needle
    - Cats: blood collection bag specifically for feline patients containing an anticoagulant, such as CPD, CPDA or ACD, attached to an extension tube and needle OR two or three 20–30 ml syringes prefilled with anticoagulant (1 ml CPD, CPDA or ACD per 7 ml blood), and a 19 or 21 G butterfly catheter and extension tubing
- 500 ml bag of crystalloid fluids and intravenous catheter (for cats)
- Topical local anaesthetic cream (e.g. EMLA cream)
- Electronic scales (for weighing blood collection bags)
- Artery forceps
- Gauze swabs
- Clamping device and clamps
- Materials for a light neck bandage

Patient preparation and positioning

- Ensure that the donor meets the criteria listed above.
- Most dogs are able to donate blood without being sedated. Cats typically require sedation.
- Restrain dogs securely in lateral recumbency or a sitting position on a table.
- Restrain cats securely in sternal recumbency with the forelimbs over the edge of the table and head raised. Alternatively, restrain the cat in lateral recumbency with the neck outstretched.
- Apply topical local anaesthetic cream and wait approximately 20–30 minutes.
- Cats should have an intravenous catheter placed in a cephalic vein for the purpose of administering intravenous fluids following blood donation.
- Aseptic preparation (see page 167–168) is carried out on the skin overlying the jugular groove.

Collection procedure

Dogs

1. An assistant should apply pressure at the thoracic inlet to raise the jugular vein. Avoid contamination of the venepuncture site.
2. Remove the needle cap and perform venepuncture using the 16 G needle attached to the collection bag. If no flashback of blood is seen in the tubing, check needle placement and tubing for occlusion. The needle may need to be repositioned, but should not be withdrawn fully from the patient.
3. Position the bag lower than the donor to aid gravitational flow, on a set of electronic scales.
4. Periodically invert the bag to ensure adequate mixing of blood and anticoagulant.
5. The maximum canine donation volume is approximately 16–18 ml/kg. The volume of blood that should be collected into a commercial blood bag is 450 ml, with an allowable 10% variance (405–495 ml). The weight of 1 ml of canine

blood is approximately 1.053 g; therefore, the weight of an acceptable unit using one of these bags is approximately 426–521 g. When the bag is full, clamp the tubing with a pair of artery forceps and remove the needle from the jugular vein.

6. Using a gauze swab, apply pressure over the venepuncture site for 5 minutes. A light neck bandage should be applied for several hours.

7. Allow the tubing to refill with anticoagulant blood and clamp the distal (needle) end with a hand sealer clip or heat sealer. If these are not available, a knot can be tied in the line, although this is less desirable.

8. Clamp the entire length of tubing into 10 cm segments to be used for cross-matching (see page 85–86).

9. Label the bag with the product type, donor identification, date of collection, date of expiration, donor blood type, donor PCV and phlebotomist identification prior to use or storage.

10. Following donation, food and water can be offered. Activity should be restricted to lead walks only for the next 24 hours, and it is advised that a harness or lead passed under the chest is used instead of a neck collar and lead, to avoid pressure on the jugular venepuncture site.

Cats

1. An assistant should apply pressure at the thoracic inlet to raise the jugular vein. Avoid contamination of the venepuncture site.

2. Remove the needle cap and perform venepuncture using the needle attached to the collection bag. If no flashback of blood is seen in the tubing, check needle placement and tubing for occlusion. The needle may need to be repositioned, but should not be withdrawn fully from the patient. Position the collecting bag lower than the donor to aid gravitational flow and on a set of electronic scales. Periodically invert the bag to ensure adequate mixing of blood and anticoagulant.
   Alternatively, use syringes containing anticoagulant and connected to a butterfly catheter. Without removing the ➡

butterfly catheter, perform venepuncture and fill each
syringe in turn. The syringes can be rocked gently to ensure
adequate mixing of blood and anticoagulant during
collection. Invert the syringes several times after filling.

3. The maximum feline donation volume is approximately
11–13 ml/kg. The volume of blood that should be collected
into a feline commercial blood bag is 50–60 ml. The weight
of 1 ml of feline blood is approximately 1.053 g; therefore,
the weight of an acceptable unit using one of these bags is
approximately 52–63 g. When the bag is full, clamp the
tubing with a pair of artery forceps and remove the needle
from the jugular vein.

   Alternatively, if collecting blood into a syringe, remove the
   needle from the vein and cap the syringe when it contains
   the desired amount.

4. Using a gauze swab, apply pressure over the venepuncture
site for 5 minutes. A light neck bandage should be applied
for several hours.

5. If a blood collection bag is used, allow the tubing to refill
with anticoagulant blood and clamp the distal (needle) end
with a hand sealer clip or heat sealer. If these are not
available, a knot can be tied in the line, although this is less
desirable. Clamp the entire length of tubing into 10 cm
segments to be used for cross-matching (see page 85–86).

6. Label the bag or syringe with the product type, donor
identification, date of collection, date of expiration, donor
blood type, donor PCV and phlebotomist identification prior
to use or storage.

7. Following donation, cats should receive intravenous fluid
replacement in the form of 30 ml/kg of intravenous
crystalloid solution over approximately 3 hours. The feline
donor must be observed closely during recovery from
sedation/general anaesthesia and may be offered food and
water once fully awake.

Potential complications

■ Haematoma
■ Hypovolaemic shock

Storage

- Whole blood collected in a bag should be stored in a refrigerator maintained at 1–6°C with the bag in an upright position. Positioning the bag in this manner maximizes gas exchange with the red cell solution to help preserve the viability of the red blood cells during storage and following transfusion.
- Whole blood collected in a bag should be used within 28 days when collected in CPD or ACD, or within 35 days when collected in CPDA.
- Feline red blood cells collected in a syringe should be used within 5 hours.
- Whole blood can also be separated into packed red blood cells, fresh plasma, stored plasma and platelet-rich plasma concentrates. This should be done as soon as possible after collection, and plasma should be frozen within 8 hours to preserve coagulation and anticoagulation factors.

Cross-matching [1]

Indications/Use

- To determine serological compatibility between a patient and donor blood

Dogs

Cross-matching should be performed whenever:

- The recipient has been transfused previously more than 4 days prior, even if a DEA 1.1-negative donor was used
- There has been a history of a transfusion reaction
- The recipient's transfusion history is unknown
- The recipient has been previously pregnant.

Cats

Cross-matching should be performed whenever:

- The recipient requires more than one transfusion, as previously transfused blood (even though it was the same AB type) may induce antibody production against red blood cell antigens separate from the AB blood group
- The donor or recipient blood type is unknown.

Equipment

- Approximately 5 ml of blood collected in EDTA anticoagulant from both the donor and recipient
- Centrifuge
- 5 ml plain plastic tubes
- 0.9% saline
- Pipette
- Microscope slides
- Microscope

Patient preparation and positioning: see Venous blood sampling, page 36–37

Technique

1. Collect blood from the jugular vein of the donor and recipient. Approximately 5 ml of blood from each should be placed into separate EDTA tubes (see page 34). Alternatively, a sample of anticoagulated blood from the clamped donor blood tubing can be used.
2. Centrifuge the tubes (usually at 1000 RPM for 5–10 minutes), remove the supernatants (plasma) and transfer them to clean labelled 5 ml plain tubes (donor and recipient) for later use.
3. If a centrifuge is not available, allow the EDTA tubes to stand for ≥1 hour until the red blood cells have settled before using the supernatant.

Standard cross-match procedure

1. Wash the red blood cells three times with 0.9% saline and discard the supernatant after each wash.
2. Resuspend the washed red blood cells to create a 3–5% solution by adding 0.2 ml of red blood cells to 4.8 ml of saline (1 drop of red blood cells to 20 drops of saline).
3. For each donor prepare three tubes labelled as major, minor and recipient control.
4. Add to each tube 1 drop of the appropriate 3–5% red blood cells and 2 drops of plasma according to the following:
   a. Major cross-match = donor red blood cells and recipient plasma

   b. Minor cross-match = recipient red blood cells and
     donor plasma

   c. Recipient control = recipient red blood cells and
     recipient plasma.

5. Incubate the tubes for 15 minutes at room temperature.

6. Centrifuge the tubes at 1000 RPM for approximately 15
   seconds to allow the cells to settle. Examine the samples for
   haemolysis (reddening of the supernatant).

7. Gently tap the tubes to resuspend the cells. Examine and
   score the tubes for agglutination.

8. If macroscopic agglutination is not
   observed, transfer a small amount of
   the tube contents to a labelled glass
   slide and examine for microscopic
   agglutination. This should not be
   confused with rouleaux formation.

Agglutination

9. For the recipient control:

   a. If there is no haemolysis or agglutination in
     the recipient control tube, the results are
     valid and incompatibilities can be interpreted

   b. If there is haemolysis or agglutination
     present in the recipient control tube, then
     the compatibility and suitability of the
     donor cannot be assessed accurately.

Rouleau

Rapid slide cross-match procedure

An alternative and more rapid, but potentially less accurate,
procedure for cross-match analysis involves visualizing the
presence of agglutination on a slide rather than in a tube

1. For each donor prepare three slides labelled as major,
   minor and recipient control.

2. Place 1 drop of red blood cells and 2 drops of plasma on to
   each slide according to the following:

   a. Major cross-match = donor red blood cells and
     recipient plasma

   b. Minor cross-match = recipient red blood cells and
     donor plasma

   c. Recipient control = recipient red blood cells and
     recipient plasma.

➡

3. Gently rock the slides to mix the plasma and red blood cells. Examine for agglutination after 1–5 minutes.
4. For the recipient control: agglutination will invalidate results.

Results of cross-matching

- Any agglutination and/or haemolysis is a 'positive' result.
- A positive **recipient control** indicates that the patient is autoagglutinating. This makes interpretation of the test difficult, although it can be repeated with additional washing of the recipient's red blood cells.
- A positive **major cross-match** indicates a significant antibody titre in the recipient against the donor red blood cells and precludes the use of that donor for transfusions.
- A positive **minor cross-match** indicates the presence of antibodies in the donor against the recipient red blood cells. If this reaction is strong, even small volumes of donor plasma may cause a significant transfusion reaction and precludes the use of the donor (unless red blood cells can be washed). With a weaker reaction, packed red blood cells from the donor may be transfused.

Despite using blood products from a cross-match-compatible donor, it is still possible for a patient to experience a haemolytic or non-haemolytic transfusion reaction. Recipient monitoring during and following administration of blood products is essential.

NOTES

Blood typing[1]

Indications/Use
- Dogs: As DEA 1.1 is the most antigenic blood type, it is strongly advised that the DEA 1.1 status of both the donor and recipient is determined prior to transfusion, or that only DEA 1.1-negative donors are used
- Cats: **All donor and recipient cats must be blood typed** prior to transfusion, even in an emergency situation

Equipment
- Approximately 2 ml of blood collected into an EDTA tube (see page 34)
- Blood typing test kit

Patient preparation and positioning: see Venous blood sampling, page 36–37

Technique
Use a commercial blood typing test kit and follow manufacturer's instructions.

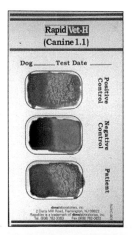

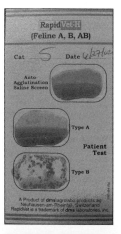

Care should be taken when blood typing severely anaemic dogs and cats. The *prozone effect* (due to the low number of red blood cells, the quantity of antigen is reduced compared with the amount of antibody in the reagent) may prevent proper agglutination of blood with the reagent. It may be helpful to centrifuge the whole blood sample and remove one drop of the plasma, to increase the relative concentration of red blood cells. The red blood cells and plasma are then remixed prior to performing the blood typing test.

Despite using blood products from a blood-typed donor, it is still possible for a patient to experience a haemolytic or non-haemolytic transfusion reaction. Recipient monitoring during and following administration of blood products is essential.

Administering the blood[1]

Indications/Use
- Anaemia due to:
  - Haemorrhage
  - Haemolysis
  - Reduced erythropoiesis

Contraindications
- Administration of non-typed or non-cross-matched blood to a dog that has previously received a blood transfusion
- Administration of non-typed blood to a cat

Equipment
As required for intravenous catheter placement
- Whole blood:
  - Dogs: As a general rule:
    - DEA 1.1-negative dogs should *only* receive DEA 1.1-negative blood

- DEA 1.1-positive dogs may receive *either* DEA 1.1-negative or -positive blood
  - Cats:
    - Type A cats must *only* receive type A blood
    - Type B cats must *only* receive type B blood
    - The rarer type AB cats do not possess either alloantibody; they should ideally receive type AB blood, but when this is not available type A blood is the next best choice
- Dogs: Blood infusion set incorporating an in-line filter (170–260 μm) and suitable for connecting to a canine blood collection bag
- Cats: Blood infusion set incorporating an in-line filter (170–260 μm) and suitable for connecting to a feline blood collection bag. Alternatively, blood collected in a syringe can be administered via an extension set. Again a filter should be used, such as a paediatric filter with reduced dead space or microaggregate filters of 18–40 μm
- Intravenous catheter suitable for the size of the patient. A large-diameter catheter should be placed to avoid red cell haemolysis during blood administration
- Adhesive tape

Patient preparation and positioning

- The patient should ideally be conscious, although sedation can be used if required. It is sometimes necessary to give blood to an anaesthetized patient intraoperatively.
- The patient should be placed on comfortable bedding and confined to a cage during the administration of blood.
- Patients should not receive food or medication during a transfusion, and the only fluid that may be administered through the same catheter is 0.9% saline.
- An intravenous catheter should be placed. *Alternatively,* blood can be given via an intraosseous needle if venous access cannot be obtained.

Technique

Blood is usually administered intravenously via an intravenous catheter, but it may also be given via the intraosseous route if venous access cannot be obtained (e.g. kittens, puppies). It should *not* be given intraperitoneally.

 Care should be taken if blood is administered to patients with increased risk of volume overload (e.g. cardiovascular disease, impaired renal function).

Volume

The amount of blood to be administered can be calculated as follows:

- As a 'rule of thumb':
  - 2 ml blood/kg bodyweight raises the PCV by 1%
- Suggested formulae for calculating the amount of whole blood required for transfusion are:
  - ### Dog:
    Volume of donor blood required =
    $$\text{recipient's bodyweight (kg)} \times 85 \times \frac{\text{desired PCV} - \text{recipient's PCV}}{\text{PCV of donated blood}}$$
  - ### Cat:
    Volume of donor blood required =
    $$\text{recipient's bodyweight (kg)} \times 60 \times \frac{\text{desired PCV} - \text{recipient's PCV}}{\text{PCV of donated blood}}$$

Total volume given should not exceed 22 ml/kg unless there are severe ongoing losses.

Rate

The rate of whole blood administration depends on the cardiovascular status of the recipient:

- In general, the rate should be only 0.25–1.0 ml/kg/h for the first 20–30 minutes
- If the transfusion is well tolerated, the rate may then be increased to deliver the remaining product within 4–6 hours

- In an animal with an increased risk of volume overload (cardiovascular disease, impaired renal function), the rate of administration should not exceed 3–4 ml/kg/h.

Monitoring

The following parameters should be measured prior to ('baseline'), every 15–30 minutes during, and 1, 12 and 24 hours after transfusion:

- Demeanour
- Rectal temperature
- Pulse rate and quality
- Respiratory rate and character
- Mucous membrane colour and capillary refill time
- Plasma and urine colour.

PCV and TP should also be monitored prior to, upon completion of, and at 12 and 24 hours after transfusion.

Adverse reactions[1]

Acute haemolytic reaction with intravascular haemolysis

- Seen in type B cats receiving type A blood as well as in DEA 1.1-negative dogs sensitized to DEA 1.1 upon repeated exposure.
- Clinical signs may include fever, tachycardia, dyspnoea, muscle tremors, vomiting, weakness, collapse, haemoglobinaemia and haemoglobinuria.
- May lead to shock, disseminated intravascular coagulation, renal damage and, potentially, death.
- **Treatment involves immediate discontinuation of the transfusion** and treatment of the clinical signs of shock.

Non-haemolytic immunological reactions

- Acute type I hypersensitivity reactions (allergic or anaphylactic), most often mediated by IgE and mast cells.
- Clinical signs may include urticaria, pruritus, erythema, oedema, vomiting and dyspnoea secondary to pulmonary oedema.

■ **Treatment involves immediate discontinuation of the transfusion** and evaluation of the patient for evidence of haemolysis and shock. Steroids (dexamethasone 0.5–1.0 mg/kg i.v.) and antihistamines (chlorphenamine 4–8 mg q8h for dogs; 2–4 mg q8–12h for cats) may be required.

NOTES

NOTES

NOTES

PART 6

Imaging

Radiographic positioning [6]

Lateral view of the pelvis

Beam centring

Over greater femoral trochanter.

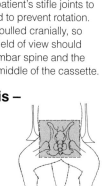

Positioning and collimation

Place into lateral recumbency with the side of interest closest to the cassette. Place foam wedge between patient's stifle joints to keep the femurs parallel to the cassette and to prevent rotation. The limb closest to the cassette should be pulled cranially, so that the femurs can be distinguished. The field of view should include entire pelvis and a portion of the lumbar spine and the femurs. Ensure the pelvis is centred to the middle of the cassette.

Ventrodorsal view of the pelvis – frog leg projection

Beam centring

Over level of pubis and acetabulum.

Positioning and collimation

The 'frog leg' view is suitable if pelvic trauma is suspected. Minimal stress and tension are placed on the pelvis and joints.

➡

Patient is in dorsal recumbency, placed in a trough. The femurs should be at a 45° angle; it is important for the femurs to be positioned identically to maintain symmetry.

Ventrodorsal view of the pelvis – extended projection

Beam centring

Over level of pubis and acetabulum.

Positioning and collimation

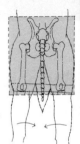

Standard evaluation for hip dysplasia. Position as for frog leg except that the hindlimbs are extended caudally, with the stifles 2.5–5 cm from each other. Secure the stifles with Velcro or ties, and secure metatarsals with sandbags.

The following criteria must be met:

- Femurs are parallel
- Both patellas are centred between the femoral condyles
- Pelvis is without rotation; obturator foramens, hip joints, hemipelvis and sacroiliac joints appear as a mirror image
- Tail is secured with tape between the femurs
- Field of view includes pelvis, femurs and stifle joints

Lateral view of the femur

Beam centring

Middle of femur.

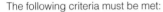

Positioning and collimation

Place into lateral recumbency with the affected limb closest to the cassette. Opposite limb is abducted and rotated out of the line of the X-ray beam. Place foam pad under the proximal tibia to alleviate any rotation of the femur. Field of view includes hip joint, femur and stifle joint.

Craniocaudal view of the femur

Beam centring

Middle of femur.

Positioning and collimation

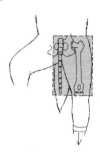

Place into dorsal recumbency with limb of
interest extended caudally. Slight
abduction of affected limb will eliminate
superimposition of the proximal femur over
the tuber ischium. The opposite limb is
flexed and rotated laterally to facilitate
abduction. The patella should be between
the two femoral condyles. Field of view
includes hip joint, femur and stifle joint.

Lateral view of the stifle

Beam centring

Over stifle joint.

Positioning and collimation

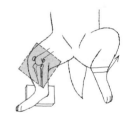

Place into lateral recumbency with the
affected joint next to the cassette.
The opposite limb is flexed and
abducted from the line of the X-ray
beam. The stifle joint should be in a natural, slightly flexed
position. Place pad under the tarsus so that the tibia is parallel to
cassette. Elevation of the tibia will ensure superimposition of the
two femoral condyles and facilitate a true lateral projection.

NOTES

Caudocranial view of the stifle

Beam centring

Over stifle joint, distal end of the femur.

Positioning and collimation

Place into sternal recumbency with
affected limb in maximum extension.
Opposite limb is flexed and elevated with
foam wedge. This will control the lateral rotation
of the stifle joint. The patella should be centred between
the femoral condyles (which can be palpated).

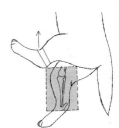

Lateral view of the tibia and fibula

Beam centring

Middle of the tibia and fibula.

Positioning and collimation

Place into lateral recumbency with the
affected limb placed on the cassette.
The stifle should be flexed slightly and
maintained in a true lateral position.
A sponge wedge can be placed under
the metatarsus to eliminate any rotation of the tibia.
The opposite limb is pulled cranially or caudally so that it is out of
the line of the beam. Field of view includes stifle joint, tibia and
fibula, and tarsal joint.

NOTES

Caudocranial view of the tibia and fibula

Beam centring

Middle of the tibia and fibula.

Positioning and collimation

Place into sternal recumbency with
the affected limb extended caudally.
Support the body with foam blocks placed
beneath the caudal abdomen and pelvic region.
Elevating the hind end will minimize the weight placed
on the stifle joint extended caudally and will facilitate
positioning. The tibia/fibula should be in a true caudocranial
position so that the patella is placed between the two femoral
condyles. Opposite limb is flexed and placed on a pad to control
rotation of the affected limb. Secure tail out of beam. Field of
view includes the stifle joint, tibia and fibula, and tarsal joint.

Lateral view of the tarsus

Beam centring

Middle of tarsus.

Positioning and collimation

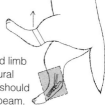

Place into lateral recumbency with affected limb
next to cassette. Tarsus is placed in a natural
slightly flexed position. The opposite limb should
be pulled cranially out of line of the X-ray beam.

NOTES

Plantarodorsal view of the tarsus

Beam centring

Middle of the tarsal joint.

Positioning and collimation

Place into sternal recumbency with
the affected limb extended as for the
caudocranial view of the tibia/fibula. Place
foam under the caudal abdomen and pelvic
region to prevent tarsal rotation. Foam also
under the stifle joint to achieve maximum extension
of the tarsus. If stifle is in true caudocranial position the tarsus
will naturally follow in a true plantarodorsal position.

Caudocranial view of the scapula

Beam centring

Middle of scapula.

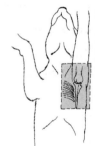

Positioning and collimation

Place in dorsal recumbency with both
forelimbs extended cranially. Sternum
rotated away from the scapula (approx.
10–20°). This avoids superimposing ribs.
Should be a clear, unobstructed view.
Collimate proximal humerus to 11th rib.

Lateral view of the shoulder

Beam centring

To shoulder joint.

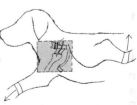

Positioning and collimation

Affected limb lowermost, patient
in lateral recumbency. Leg is
extended cranial and ventral to

sternum to prevent superimposition. Other leg is pulled in a caudodorsal (CdD) direction. The neck is extended dorsally. Sternum is rotated slightly. Collimate mid-scapula to mid-humerus.

Caudocranial view of the shoulder

Beam centring

To shoulder joint.

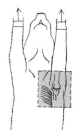

Positioning and collimation

Place in dorsal recumbency with both forelimbs extended cranially until parallel with cassette. *Caution: do not rotate humerus.* Collimate mid-humerus, and two-thirds along scapula.

Lateral view of the humerus

Beam centring

Centre of humerus.

Positioning and collimation

Place in lateral recumbency with affected limb lowermost. Extend in cranioventral (CrV) direction with the opposite limb drawn in a CdD direction. Head and neck should be extended dorsally. Collimate mid-radius/ulna and distal end of scapula.

Flexed lateral view of the elbow

Beam centring

Middle of elbow.

Positioning and collimation

Place in lateral recumbency with affected limb lowermost. Carpus is pulled toward the neck region, flexing the elbow.

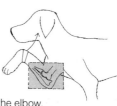

➡

Care should be taken to keep elbow in true lateral position during flexion. By keeping the carpus lateral, the elbow should also remain in a true lateral position.

Lateral view of the elbow

Beam centring

Over elbow joint.

Positioning and collimation

Place in lateral recumbency with affected limb lowermost. Slightly extend the head and neck in a dorsal direction and the unaffected limb in a caudodorsal direction. Place foam wedge under the metacarpal region to maintain a true lateral view of the elbow.

Craniocaudal view of the elbow

Beam centring

Over elbow joint.

Positioning and collimation

Place in sternal recumbency with the affected limb extended cranially. Elevate patient's head and position away from affected side. Exact view will provide the olecranon between the medial and lateral humeral epicondyles. Place foam pad under point of elbow to prevent rolling or rotation.

Lateral view of the radius and ulna

Beam centring

Middle of radius and ulna.

Positioning and collimation

Place in lateral recumbency with affected limb centred on cassette. The opposite limb is drawn caudally

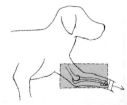

out of the way. The primary X-ray beam should include the elbow and carpal joints.

Craniocaudal view of the radius and ulna

Beam centring

Middle of radius and ulna.

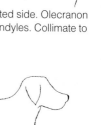

Positioning and collimation

Place in sternal recumbency with affected limb extended cranially.

Elevate head and position away from affected side. Olecranon should be placed between the humeral condyles. Collimate to include the elbow and the carpus.

Lateral view of the carpus

Beam centring

Over distal row of carpal bones.

Positioning and collimation

Place in lateral recumbency with affected limb in centre of cassette.

Place foam wedge under elbow to prevent carpus moving away from cassette. Other leg is pulled caudally out of the way. Flexed lateral can be obtained in this position also. Collimate to include distal radius/ulna, whole of carpus and proximal end of metacarpals.

NOTES

Dorsopalmar view of the carpus

Beam centring

Middle of distal row of carpal bones.

Positioning and collimation

Place in sternal recumbency with affected limb extended cranially. Carpus is flat against cassette. Place foam wedge under elbow. Oblique views are obtained with 45° angle of the dorsopalmar view to provide dorsopalmar mediolateral (DPaML) and dorsopalmar lateromedial (DPaLM) views. Stress views are with the carpus in dorsopalmar (DPa) position, with radius and ulna firmly held in place. Paw is pushed medially or laterally with a ruler or a wooden paddle. Do not apply *too* much stress. Collimate to include entire carpus with two-thirds of the metacarpals and the distal end of the radius/ulna.

Lateral view of the phalangeal isolation

Beam centring

Centre of digit.

Positioning and collimation

Place in lateral recumbency with affected side adjacent to cassette. Place a foam pad under the elbow to alleviate rotation. Superimposition is a problem here: if one digit is to be examined, isolate from the other digits by taping it cranially in a fixed position; a further band of tape can be used to hold the remaining digits back. Collimate distal ulna/radius and entire paw.

Lateral view of the skull

Beam centring

Lateral canthus of eye.

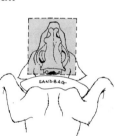

Positioning and collimation

Place into lateral recumbency with affected side next to cassette. Place a foam wedge under the ramus of the mandible to stop rotation. The nasal septum should be parallel to the cassette. Place another wedge under the CrV cervical region; pull the front limbs caudally. Field of view should include the tip of the nose to the base of the skull.

Dorsoventral view of the skull

Beam centring

Lateral canthus of eye, over high point of cranium.

Positioning and collimation

Place into sternal recumbency with the head resting on the cassette. A sandbag should be placed gently over the cervical region to help gain a true dorsoventral (DV) position. Keep the forelimbs in a natural position alongside the head, but out of the beam. The sagittal plane of the head should be perpendicular. Tape over the cranium can be used to secure this position. Field of view includes tip of nose to base of skull.

Ventrodorsal view of the skull

Beam centring

Lateral canthus of eye, midline mandibular rami.

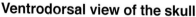

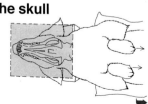

Positioning and collimation

Place into dorsal recumbency. A trough or sandbags can be used to keep animal in position. The front limbs are extended caudally and secured. A foam pad should be placed under the mid-cervical region to gain proper positioning of the skull on the cassette. The nose must remain parallel to the cassette, and the skull must be balanced in a true ventrodorsal (VD) position. Place a small pad under the cranium to prevent rotation, if needed. Field of view includes the tip of the nose to the base of skull.

Rostrocaudal view of the frontal sinuses

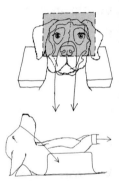

Beam centring

Through centre of frontal sinuses between eyes.

Positioning and collimation

Place into dorsal recumbency with the nose pointing upwards. Pull forelimbs caudally alongside the body. Nose is positioned

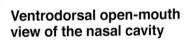

perpendicular to cassette. Apply a tie around the nose to stabilize. A tongue clamp may also be used to help secure, if needed. Field of view includes the entire forehead of the patient.

Ventrodorsal open-mouth view of the nasal cavity

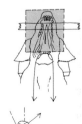

Beam centring

Through level of third upper premolar. To centre on nasal cavity.

Positioning and collimation

Place into dorsal recumbency, extending forelimbs caudally alongside the body. Keep the maxilla parallel to the cassette and secure with a tie or tape. Tie the endotracheal tube to the mandible. Apply a tie around the mandible and pull in a caudal direction to open the mouth (a tongue clamp may also be used, also being secured caudally). Angle the tube head to 10–15°, to direct into the mouth. Field of view should include the entire maxilla from the tip of the nose to the pharyngeal region.

Open-mouth lateral oblique view of the lower dental arcade

Beam centring

Over site of interest.

Positioning and collimation

Place into lateral recumbency with affected mandible next to the cassette. Place a radiolucent gag into the mouth, to separate the upper and lower jaws. Rotate the cranium approx. 20° away from the tabletop and maintain this position with a foam wedge.

Ventrodorsal intraoral view of the mandible

Beam centring

Over site of interest.

Positioning and collimation

Place into dorsal recumbency. Extend the head cranially. Place a non-screen film into the mouth with the corner edge of the film introduced first. Advance until the lips allow no further. Pull the tongue cranially to eliminate uneven density over the mandibular area. Because the source-to-image distance is reduced (as the film is elevated from the table), the X-ray tube should be raised to compensate.

Open-mouth ventrodorsal oblique view of the upper dental arcade

Beam centring

Over third premolar.

Positioning and collimation

Place the patient halfway on to its back with the maxillary arcade of interest closest to the cassette. Rotate the head approx. 45° to the cassette, and stabilize on a foam wedge. The rotation prevents superimposition. Maintain the mouth open with use of a radiolucent mouth gag or by securing the mandible back, with the tongue being pulled back by a tongue depressor.

Dorsoventral intraoral view of the maxilla

Beam centring

Over site of interest.

Positioning and collimation

Place into sternal recumbency with the head kept in line with the spine. Place a non-screen film into the mouth, and advance caudally between the lips. The X-ray tube should be elevated to compensate for the reduction in source-to-image distance.

Lateral oblique view of the tympanic bullae

Beam centring

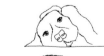

Over centre of tympanic bullae.

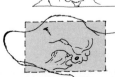

Positioning and collimation

Place into lateral recumbency with unaffected tympanic bulla toward the cassette. The forelimbs are extended slightly caudally. The skull should lie naturally at 8–12° rotation from true lateral. This causes the tympanic bullae to lie separately, allowing visualization of a single bulla. This view can also be used to examine an oblique projection of the temporomandibular joints.

Rostrocaudal open-mouth view of the tympanic bullae

Beam centring

At level of commissure of lips.

Positioning and collimation

Place into dorsal recumbency with nose pointing upwards and forelimbs pulled caudally, along the body. Secure the mouth open with ties and tongue clamp, and pull caudally. Pull the nose 5–10° cranially, pulling the mandible caudally. The bullae should be projected free from the mandible and the hard palate of the maxilla. Field of view includes the entire nasopharyngeal region of the skull.

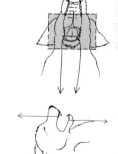

NOTES

Rostrocaudal view of the cranium

Beam centring

Midpoint between eyes.

Positioning and collimation

Place into dorsal recumbency with the nose pointing upwards and forelimbs pulled caudally alongside the body. Angle the nose slightly caudally (approx. 10–15°). A tie around the nose (± tongue clamp) may be used to secure this position. Field of view includes the entire cranium. *Warning: ensure endotracheal tube does not kink.*

Ventrodorsal oblique view of the temporomandibular joint (TMJ)

Beam centring

Over centre of TMJ.

Positioning and collimation

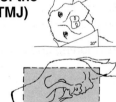

Place in lateral recumbency with affected side next to the cassette. Rotate the cranium 20° towards the cassette. Place a sponge wedge under the mandible to secure the skull into position. This rotation will help prevent superimposition. This view can be taken with or without the mouth open.

NOTES

Flexed lateral view of the cervical spine

Beam centring

C3–4 intervertebral space.

Positioning and collimation

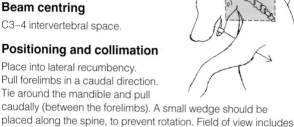

Place into lateral recumbency.
Pull forelimbs in a caudal direction.
Tie around the mandible and pull
caudally (between the forelimbs). A small wedge should be placed along the spine, to prevent rotation. Field of view includes base of skull and first few thoracic vertebrae. *Warning: care must be taken not to bend the endotracheal tube causing a blockage, or further traumatize the spine (i.e. atlanto-axial subluxation).*

Extended lateral view of the cervical spine

Beam centring

Intervertebral space of C4 and C5.

Positioning and collimation

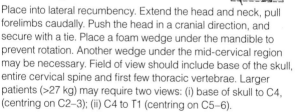

Place into lateral recumbency. Extend the head and neck, pull forelimbs caudally. Push the head in a cranial direction, and secure with a tie. Place a foam wedge under the mandible to prevent rotation. Another wedge under the mid-cervical region may be necessary. Field of view should include base of the skull, entire cervical spine and first few thoracic vertebrae. Larger patients (>27 kg) may require two views: (i) base of skull to C4, (centring on C2–3); (ii) C4 to T1 (centring on C5–6).

NOTES

Ventrodorsal view of the cervical spine

Beam centring

Over C4–5 intervertebral space.

Positioning and collimation

Place into dorsal recumbency. Extend the
head cranially and pull forelimbs cranially
along the body. Place a small wedge under
the mid-cervical region to eliminate any distortion. Field of view
includes the base of the skull, entire cervical spine and the first
few thoracic vertebrae. Larger patients (>27 kg) may require two
views: (i) base of skull to C4 (centring on C2–3); (ii) C4 to T1
(centring on C56).

Lateral view of the thoracic spine

Beam centring

Over 7th thoracic vertebral body.

Positioning and collimation

Place into lateral recumbency. Extend
forelimbs cranially and hindlimbs caudally. Place a wedge under
the sternum so that the sternum is at the same height as the
thoracic vertebrae. Field of view includes the area from the 7th
cervical vertebral body to the 1st lumbar vertebral body.

NOTES

Ventrodorsal view of the thoracic spine

Beam centring

Over level of caudal border of scapula.

Positioning and collimation

Place into dorsal recumbency. Extend
forelimbs cranially. Allow hindlimbs to lie
naturally. The sternum should superimpose
the thoracic spine; a trough may be required. Field of view
includes all the thoracic vertebrae from C7 to L1.

Lateral view of the thoracolumbar spine

Beam centring

Over thoracolumbar junction.

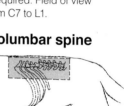

Positioning and collimation

Place into lateral recumbency.
Extend forelimbs cranially and hindlimbs caudally. Place a
wedge under the sternum to bring it level to the spine. Field of
view includes the entire thoracolumbar spine.

Ventrodorsal view of the thoracolumbar spine

Beam centring

Over thoracolumbar junction.

Positioning and collimation

Place into dorsal recumbency. Extend
forelimbs cranially. Hindlimbs can lie in their
natural position. Superimpose the sternum
with the thoracic vertebrae; a trough can be used. Field of view
includes all the thoracic and lumbar vertebrae.

Lateral view of the lumbar spine

Beam centring

Over level of 4th lumbar
vertebral body.

Positioning and collimation

Place into lateral recumbency.
Extend the forelimbs cranially and hindlimbs caudally.
Place foam wedges under the sternum, mid-lumbar region and
between the hindlimbs to prevent rotation. Field of view is from
the 13th thoracic vertebral body to 1st sacral vertebral body.

Ventrodorsal view of the lumbar spine

Beam centring

Over 4th lumbar vertebral body.

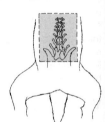

Positioning and collimation

Place into dorsal recumbency with
forelimbs extended cranially. Allow
hindlimbs to lie in natural position;
wedges may be placed under the
stifles and use a trough to stabilize.
Field of view includes the entire lumbar spine from the 13th
thoracic vertebral body to the 1st sacral vertebral body.

Lateral view of the pharynx

Beam centring

Over pharynx.

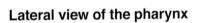

Positioning and collimation

Place into lateral recumbency. Extend forelimbs
caudally. Extend head and neck cranially. Place a wedge
under the mandible, to help prevent rotation. The upper
respiratory tract passages act as a negative contrast agent

allowing the structures of the pharynx to be visible. Field of view includes the entire area of the neck between the lateral canthus of the eye and the 3rd cervical vertebral body.

Lateral view of the thorax

Beam centring

Over caudal border of scapula.

Positioning and collimation

Place into right lateral recumbency –
this provides the most accurate view of the cardiac silhouette. If lung metastases are suspected, both right and left views should be obtained for any subtle changes. Extend forelimbs cranially; this helps reduce superimposition of the triceps and humeri over the cranial aspect of the thorax. Extend hindlimbs slightly caudally. Extend the head slightly. Place a wedge under the mandible and thorax, and between the hindlimbs, to prevent rotation. Field of view includes the entire thoracic cavity from the line of the manubrium sterni caudally to the 1st lumbar vertebral body. Exposure is taken at full inspiration.

Ventrodorsal view of the thorax

Beam centring

Over caudal border of scapula.

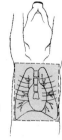

Positioning and collimation

This view allows full visualization of the lung fields, providing better views of the accessory lung lobe and caudal mediastinum. Place into dorsal recumbency. Extend forelimbs cranially. Hindlimbs stay as normal. Superimpose the sternum with the spine. Use of a trough may help secure the position. Exposure is taken at full inspiration.

This view is contraindicated in patients with respiratory problems.

Dorsoventral view of the thorax

Beam centring

Over caudal border of scapula.

Positioning and collimation

DV is best for the evaluation of the heart, because the heart is nearer the sternum and it sits in its normal position. This position is difficult for deep-chested breeds; use plenty of wedges and positioning aids; if unable to do, VD will have to be taken.

Place into sternal recumbency. Superimpose the spine over the sternum. Extend forelimbs slightly cranially to keep elbows out of view. Hindlimbs are as normal (difficult for hip dysplastic dogs). Lower the head and place between the two forelimbs. Field of view includes the entire thorax, including all ribs. The exposure should be taken at full inspiration, to allow complete visualization of the lung tissue.

Lateral view of the abdomen

Beam centring

Over caudal aspect of 13th rib (for feline, measure 2–3 fingerbreadths caudally).

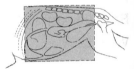

Positioning and collimation

Place into right lateral recumbency. Extend hindlimbs caudally. The right view facilitates longitudinal separation of the kidneys. Extend the hindlimbs caudally to prevent superimposition of the femoral muscles over the caudal portion of the abdomen. Place a pad between the femurs to prevent rotation of the pelvis and caudal abdomen. A pad should also be placed under the sternum, to keep sternum at the same level as the spine. Field of view includes the diaphragm caudally to the femoral head. Take the exposure at the time of expiration so that the diaphragm is displaced cranially.

Ventrodorsal view of the abdomen

Beam centring

Over caudal aspect of 13th rib (for feline measure 2–3 fingerbreadths caudally).

Positioning and collimation

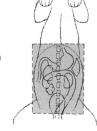

Place into dorsal recumbency. Use a trough or sandbags for positioning. Field of view includes the entire abdomen from the diaphragm to the level of the femoral head. Larger patients may require two views: one of the cranial abdomen and the other of the caudal abdomen. Take exposure during the expiratory phase so that the diaphragm is in a cranial position and not placing any compression on the abdominal contents.

Advanced radiographic positioning[2]

Feline tympanic bulla

View

- Rostral 10° ventral–caudodorsal oblique (R10°V–CdDO) view

Beam centring

Centre in the midline over the pharynx, just caudal to the ramus of the mandible.

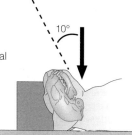

Positioning and collimation

Place the cat in dorsal recumbency supported in a trough. Secure forelimbs caudally with sandbags. Flex the head so that the hard palate is positioned 10° beyond the vertical and support in position using a foam wedge.

Comments

This view enables visualization of the tympanic bullae whilst keeping the mouth closed. It is a useful alternative to the open-mouth rostrocaudal (RCd) view, especially in cats. It is important to make sure the head and body are kept in a straight line. Make sure the anaesthetic circuit is supported adequately while performing this view.

Temporomandibular joint (TMJ)

Views

- Left lateral 20° rostral–right lateral caudal oblique (Lt20°R–RtCdO) (closed mouth) view
- Right lateral 20° rostral–left lateral caudal oblique (Rt20°R–LtCdO) (closed mouth) view

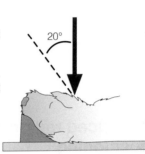

Beam centring

Centre on the caudoventral border of the uppermost zygomatic arch at the level of the external ear canal.

Positioning and collimation

Place the patient in lateral recumbency with the side under examination closer to the cassette. Place head in true lateral recumbency, with the hard palate positioned perpendicular to the cassette. Elevate the nose between 10° and 30° to the cassette with a triangular foam wedge:

- Dolichocephalic breeds – 10°
- Mesaticephalic breeds – 15°
- Brachycephalic breeds – 20–30°

Collimate to include the area of interest.

Comments

This view allows the TMJ to be visualized without superimposition of other structures. By raising the patient's nose, the TMJ adjacent to the cassette is highlighted rostrally and should be labelled L or R as appropriate. When investigating jaw-locking or TMJ pain, these views should be repeated with the mouth open.

Limbs

Carpus (1)

View

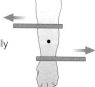

- Dorsopalmar (DPa) laterally and medially stressed views

Beam centring

Centre in the midline at the level of the antebrachiocarpal joint.

Positioning and collimation

Place the patient in sternal recumbency with the head supported on a foam pad to reduce rotation. Extend the forelimb under investigation cranially and secure it, using foam wedges and sandbags to prevent rotation.

Medial distraction: Place adhesive tape or a tie around the distal radius/ulna proximal to the carpus (without obscuring any of the carpal bones). Secure the tape medially (a sandbag may be useful). Place a second piece of tape around the foot and distract the distal limb laterally and secure it in the same way. Collimate to include the distal third of the radius/ulna and the foot.

Lateral distraction: Repeat as for the medial distraction view but reverse the tapes.

Comments

These stressed views are used when collateral joint instability is suspected. They can also be used to highlight suspected carpal fractures but care must be taken not to cause additional fracture displacement. It is important to include the foot as this will help to visualize the degree of laxity in the joint. Markers should be used at the level of each tape to identify the direction of forces used to stress the joint.

➥

Carpus (2)

Views

- Mediolateral extended (ML extended) view

- Mediolateral flexed (ML flexed) view

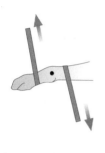

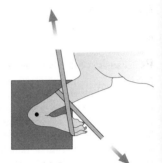

Beam centring

Centre at the level of the antebrachiocarpal joint.

Positioning and collimation

Place the patient in lateral recumbency with the limb under investigation adjacent to the cassette. The other limb should be secured caudally using a tie. Using the adhesive tapes or ties proximal and distal to the carpal joint, the carpus should be secured in maximum extension for the extended view, and in maximum flexion for the flexed view. Collimate to include the distal third of the radius/ulna and the foot.

Comments

Including the foot helps to visualize the degree of laxity in the joint.

Tarsus (1)

View

- Plantarodorsal (PID) laterally/medially stressed views

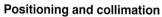

Beam centring

Centre in the midline at the level of the tibiotarsal joint.

Positioning and collimation

Place the patient in sternal recumbency with the head supported on a foam pad. Place padding under the hindlimb not under investigation. This helps to rotate the pelvis so that the limb of interest can be fully extended caudally. Apply adhesive tapes or ties proximal and distal to the tarsal joint, distracting the proximal limb medially and the distal limb laterally. Collimate to include the distal third of the tibia and the foot. Reverse the tapes to distract the joint medially.

Comments

Markers should be used at the level of each tape to identify the direction of forces used to stress the joint.

Tarsus (2)

Views

- Mediolateral extended (ML extended) view

- Mediolateral flexed (ML flexed) view

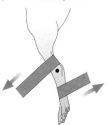
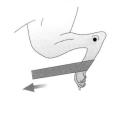

➥

Beam centring

Centre at the level of the tibiotarsal joint.

Positioning and collimation

Place the patient in lateral recumbency with the limb under investigation adjacent to the cassette. The other limb should be secured out of the way using a tie. Apply the adhesive tape or a tie proximal and distal to the tarsal joint and secure the joint in maximum extension or in maximum flexion as required. Collimate to include the distal third of the tibia and the foot.

Comments

Including the foot helps to visualize the degree of laxity in the joint.

Shoulder

View

- Cranioproximal–craniodistal oblique (CrPr–CrDiO) flexed skyline view

Beam centring

Centre over the bicipital groove between the greater and lesser tuberosities of the humerus.

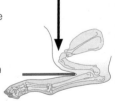

Positioning and collimation

Place the patient in sternal recumbency, with the head supported on a foam pad and rotated away from the shoulder to be radiographed. The sternum should also be rotated slightly away from the shoulder. Pads placed under the opposite forelimb may help with positioning. The limb under investigation needs to be fully flexed and the carpus brought caudally so that it is under the shoulder, with the foot placed slightly medially. The elbow needs to be held close to the body, which will help to keep the humerus straight. The cassette needs to be positioned into the crease of the elbow, held in position between the humerus and radius. Collimate to include the area of interest.

Comments

This view is useful in the investigation of mineralized opacities seen on a mediolateral view, and helps to determine whether such opacities lie within the bicipital groove. It is also useful for showing any new bone formation within the groove.

Film faults[6]

Fault	Causes
Background too light	Probably underdeveloped Possibly underexposed (exposure too low) Low line voltage
Poorly penetrated 'silhouette' image	Underexposed or underdeveloped
Penetrated image with a thin background	Overexposed and underdeveloped (Underdevelopment leads to overexposure)
Background correct but image too dark	Overexposed (exposure factors too high) Fogged (chemicals, light, wrong safelight filter or bulb) White light leakage into darkroom or cassette Old film or film exposed to scatter/chemicals, pressure Over-development
Blurred image	Movement of the patient, tube head or cassette during exposure Poor screen–film contact Incorrect screen Scatter Film fogging
Film discoloured after storage	Poorly washed or poorly fixed film
White marks on the film	Dirt or scratch on the screen Scratch on film before exposure or after processing Splash of fixer on to film or greasy fingerprints before developing

➡

Fault	Causes
Black marks on the film	Scratch on film between exposure and processing Splash of developer before processing Water splash after developing Bending or pressure after exposure ('crimp marks')
High contrast	Low kV technique used
Low contrast	High kV Scatter (no grid used) Poor processing (e.g. exhausted developer)
Uneven processing	Poorly mixed chemicals Films touching during processing Poor agitation of films during processing
Black spots or lightning-like lines	Static electricity

NOTES

NOTES

NOTES

PART 7

Anaesthesia and analgesia

ASA scale of anaesthetic risk[9]

I:	A normal healthy patient – e.g. a young dog presented for elective ovariohysterectomy
II:	A patient with mild systemic disease – e.g. a dog with a low-grade heart murmur that is not showing any clinical signs of cardiac disease
III:	A patient with severe systemic disease – e.g. a dog with a heart murmur that has resulted in reduced exercise tolerance
IV:	A patient with severe systemic disease that is a constant threat to life – e.g. a dog with a cardiac arrhythmia that is causing severe circulatory compromise
V:	A moribund patient that is not expected to survive without the operation – e.g. a dog with gastric dilatation and volvulus
E:	Denotes that the procedure is an emergency

NOTES

Anaesthetic equipment

How to choose an anaesthetic breathing circuit [6,9]

T-piece

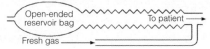

Used for *continuous* IPPV?	Yes
Fresh gas flow rate	500–600 ml/kg/min
Circuit factor	2.5–3
Patient weight range	<10 kg
Can be used with nitrous oxide?	Yes
Advantages	Lightweight, cheap, semi-disposable
Disadvantages	Difficult to scavenge from
Comments	Circuit often now sold with a plastic APL and closed reservoir bag that, although not technically a T-Piece, can be used in the same way and is easier to scavenge from

Bain

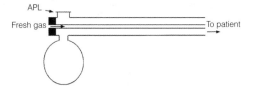

Used for *continuous* IPPV?	Yes
Fresh gas flow rate	400–500 ml/kg/min
Circuit factor	2–2.5
Patient weight range	<15–20 kg

Can be used with nitrous oxide?	Yes
Advantages	Lightweight, cheap, semi-disposable Can be used for continuous IPPV
Disadvantages	High fresh gas flow rates preclude its use in larger animals
Comments	Can be used with a ventilator to provide continuous mechanical IPPV Inner pipe can become disconnected or leak at the anaesthetic machine end, resulting in re-breathing

Lack

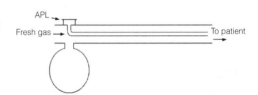

Used for *continuous* IPPV?	No
Fresh gas flow rate	160–200 ml/kg/min
Circuit factor	1–1.5
Patient weight range	>12 kg
Can be used with nitrous oxide?	Yes
Advantages	Lightweight, cheap, semi-disposable Lower flow rates than the Bain
Disadvantages	Not suitable for continuous IPPV
Comments	Inner pipe can become disconnected or leak at the anaesthetic machine end, resulting in re-breathing

Parallel Lack

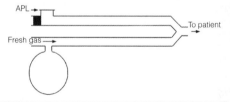

Used for *continuous* IPPV?	No
Fresh gas flow rate	160–200 ml/kg/min
Circuit factor	1–1.5
Patient weight range	>12 kg
Can be used with nitrous oxide?	Yes
Advantages	Lightweight, cheap, semi-disposable Lower flow rates than the Bain
Disadvantages	Parallel breathing pipes increase the drag on the endotracheal tube
Comments	Identical in function to the Lack Leaks or damage more easily identified

Humphrey ADE without soda lime cannister

Used for *continuous* IPPV?	Yes
Fresh gas flow rate	100–150 ml/kg/min
Circuit factor	0.5–0.75

Patient weight range	<10 kg
Can be used with nitrous oxide?	Yes
Advantages	Lower flow rates than a standard parallel Lack
Disadvantages	Suitable for continuous IPPV (and can be configured to work with a mechanical ventilator)
Comments	The special APL valve fitted to these circuits maximizes dead-space gas conservation, allowing lower flow rates to be used The APL valve design might also reduce alveolar collapse during anaesthesia

Magill

Used for *continuous* IPPV?	No
Fresh gas flow rate	160–200 ml/kg/min
Circuit factor	0.70–1
Patient weight range	>12 kg
Can be used with nitrous oxide?	Yes
Advantages	None
Disadvantages	Valve at the patient end of the circuit is difficult to scavenge
Comments	The Humphrey ADE and parallel Lack have now replaced the Magill and should be preferred

➡

Circle

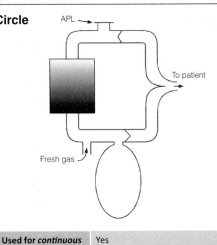

Used for *continuous* IPPV?	Yes
Fresh gas flow rate	Initially: 2–4 l/min After 5 minutes: 1–2 l/min
Circuit factor	N/A
Patient weight range	>15 kg
Can be used with nitrous oxide?	No, unless respiratory gas monitoring is available
Advantages	Low flow rates reduce costs and environmental pollution
Disadvantages	Large resistance to breathing Not suitable for short procedures
Comments	Do not use with nitrous oxide (unless respiratory gas monitoring is available) The relative positions of the fresh gas inlet, the reservoir bag and the APL valve vary between manufacturers The reservoir bag is best placed on the inspiratory limb. Circle circuits with the inspiratory bag on the expiratory limb offer a much greater resistance to inspiration

Humphrey ADE with soda lime canister

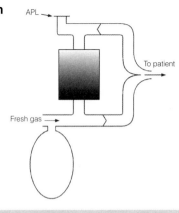

Used for *continuous* IPPV?	Yes
Fresh gas flow rate	Initially: 30 ml/kg/min After 5 minutes: 10 ml/kg/min (minimum flow 300 ml/min)
Circuit factor	N/A
Patient weight range	>7 kg
Can be used with nitrous oxide?	No, unless respiratory gas monitoring is available
Advantages	Very low flow rates achievable (a 30 kg dog requires only 300 ml/min) reducing costs and environmental pollution Lightweight valves allow it to be used on patients that would not be able to use a normal circle Made of non-ferrous metals so can be used in an MRI scanner The unique APL valve ensures that gas is conserved within the circuit even during rapid respiration
Disadvantages	Initial purchase price is high
Comments	Do not use with nitrous oxide (unless respiratory gas monitoring is available)

The Humphrey ADE circuit [6]

The Humphrey ADE circuit is a relatively new innovation in veterinary anaesthesia but it has been used in medical practice for the last two decades. It was invented by Dr Humphrey in the 1980s. Because of some of its unique design features, it can be used in animals varying in size from a cat to a Great Dane. The circuit can be used in two basic configurations: with or without soda lime.

Humphrey ADE circuit with soda lime

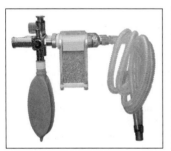 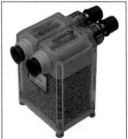

- The Humphrey ADE circuit can be fitted with a soda lime canister, making it into a small circle circuit. This can be used for animals weighing more than 7 kg.

Humphrey ADE circuit without soda lime

- Without soda lime, the circuit works like a Lack with a proportion of the dead-space gas being rebreathed.
- The narrow smooth-bore tubing means that it can be used on cats, larger birds and reptiles as well as dogs.
- The modified pop-off valve improves on the efficiency of the

normal Lack circuit, allowing lower flow rates than those recommended for a normal Lack circuit to be used safely.

'Lever' on the Humphrey ADE circuit

- The lever on the side of the Humphrey ADE circuit changes its configuration so that it can be used with a mechanical ventilator either with or without the soda lime canister.
- The lever **must** be left up, unless the circuit is connected to a ventilator.

The Humphrey APL valve[6]

The Humphrey ADE circuit is fitted with a special APL valve that contributes to the circuit's efficiency. Like a parallel Lack, it is possible to reduce the fresh gas flow used until the animal starts to rebreathe the dead-space gas from the previous breath. Of the gas exhaled by an animal, 30–40% is dead-space gas and, as it is free of carbon dioxide, it can be conserved in the breathing circuit and delivered to the patient during the next breath. In theory, the exhaled dead-space gases in a Lack and parallel Lack pass back down the inspiratory limb of the circuit until the reservoir bag is full. Then the alveolar gases pass down the expiratory limb towards the APL valve. In practice, the APL valve opens before the reservoir bag is full and some of the dead-space gas is lost.

The Humphrey APL valve is designed not to open until the reservoir bag is full, conserving more of the dead-space gas in the inspiratory limb of the circuit.

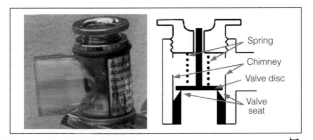

Spring
Chimney
Valve disc
Valve seat

The Humphrey APL valve has another benefit. During anaesthesia, the alveoli in the dependent (lower) lung lobes collapse and do not fill with anaesthetic gases. This reduces gas exchange and can contribute to hypoxia in patients with compromised pulmonary function. The APL valve on the Humphrey ADE circuit closes earlier in the breathing cycle, maintaining a slight positive pressure (1 cmH_2O) in the circuit and the patient's lungs. In children this has been demonstrated to prevent alveolar collapse and it is likely that the same benefit exists in small animals.

Phase 1 – Early expiration

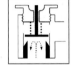

The pressure in the circuit rises and the valve disc lifts off the valve seat, but the valve effectively remains closed as the valve disc does not get pushed completely out of the valve chimney. This prevents the dead-space gas from leaving the circuit and it must all flow into the *inspiratory* limb, where it is conserved.

Phase 2 – Late expiration

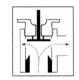

Once the reservoir bag is full the pressure in the circuit rises still further, lifting the valve disc beyond the valve chimney and allowing the alveolar gases to escape into the scavenging system.

Phase 3 – Expiratory pause

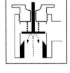

At the end of expiration the valve closes again but the valve disc falls back into the chimney at a pressure of 1 cmH_2O, preventing the last few millilitres of gas from escaping and maintaining a slight positive pressure in the circuit *and* in the patient's lungs during the expiratory pause. In children at least, this prevents alveolar collapse.

Phase 4 – Inspiration

The valve disc is held against the valve seat by the spring, preventing gas from being drawn back in from the atmosphere. This prevents carbon dioxide-rich alveolar gas now sitting in the expiratory limb from being drawn back towards the patient. The patient must breathe carbon dioxide-free dead-space gas and fresh gas from the inspiratory limb.

Calculating fresh gas flow rates[9]

Due to the reliance on the fresh gas flow rate to prevent rebreathing, correct calculation of fresh gas flow rate is essential.

1. Calculate the patient's **tidal volume** (TV). This is the volume of gas exhaled in one breath and is considered to be between 10 and 15 ml/kg.

   - The size of the patient is the first thing to consider when determining which end of the 10–15 ml/kg range to use. Generally, use the high end of the range for small dogs and cats. For larger patients, e.g. Labradors, a tidal volume of 10 ml/kg is appropriate.
   - Consider the body condition of the patient. Only the lean weight, i.e. what the bodyweight would be at a body condition score of 3/5, should be used in the calculation.
   - Consider the shape of the patient's thorax. Deep-chested breeds such as Greyhounds will have a higher tidal volume than would be expected for their bodyweight (12–15 ml/kg).

   Tidal volume (ml) **= 10–15 × bodyweight** (kg)

2. Calculate the patient's **minute volume** (MV). This is the volume of gas expired by the patient in 1 minute and requires measurement of respiratory rate (breaths per minute). This should be done when the patient has been allowed to acclimatize to its environment. The best way of gathering this information is to observe the patient from a distance when it is in its kennel. If the patient is panting, the respiratory rate should be estimated. Once the patient is anaesthetized the

➡

respiratory rate may be different to that used for the MV calculation. It is important to recalculate MV if the respiratory rate increases, as it will lead to increased MV.

Minute volume (ml/min) =
Tidal volume (ml) × **Respiratory rate** (/min)

3. Multiply the calculated minute volume by the **circuit factor** of the breathing system being used. The circuit factor varies between different breathing systems.

Fresh gas flow rate (ml/min) =
Minute volume (ml/min) × **Circuit factor**

NOTES

Checking anaesthetic equipment[7]

This procedure should be followed at the start of each working day. In addition, steps 2, 11, 16 and 20–33 should be completed prior to each new patient being connected to the system.

1. Take note of any information or labelling on the anaesthetic machine referring to the current status of the machine. Read service labels and pay attention to the last service date.
2. Check all monitoring devices are functioning and ready for use: pulse oximeter, blood pressure, capnograph (check sampling lines are attached properly and free from obstructions).
3. Ensure flowmeters are turned off.
4. Press oxygen flush valve until no gas flows through the common gas outlet.
5. Check all flowmeters and pressure gauges are at zero.
6. Ensure the reserve oxygen cylinder is connected securely to the hanger yoke.
7. Open the reserve oxygen cylinder valve slowly, anticlockwise. Take note of the registered pressure.
8. Replace the cylinder if the gas content is low.
9. Label the cylinder as 'in use' or 'full' depending on its contents.
10. Turn off the emergency cylinder and ensure the pressure gauge returns to zero.
11. Connect the Schrader probe of the piped oxygen supply to the corresponding gas supply terminal outlet, giving a gentle tug to ensure they are connected correctly. A safety alarm may sound when piped oxygen is connected and disconnected (this is a safety feature to indicate low oxygen pressure).
12. Check that the pipeline pressure gauges (if applicable) on the anaesthetic machine indicate 400 kPa (kilopascals) (4 bar).
13. Open and then close the oxygen flowmeter to ensure it is working smoothly and that the bobbin (or ball) is spinning and is not sticking to the side of the flowmeter. Check the vaporizer to ensure that it contains enough liquid anaesthetic agent; replenish if necessary, ensuring that it is not overfilled. ➡

14. Check that the vaporizer is seated correctly and locked on the back bar.
15. Adjust the control spindle on the vaporizer, ensuring it turns smoothly.
16. Turn the vaporizer to the 'off' position.
17. Check that the filling port on the vaporizer is closed correctly.
18. Select the breathing system required for use, based on the patient's bodyweight, the procedure to be performed and whether IPPV is intended.
19. Visually inspect the system for correct configuration and soiling. Replace or clean if necessary.
20. Visually inspect the patient-end tubing, ensuring no blockages are present.
21. Connect the breathing system to the common gas outlet of the anaesthetic machine.
22. Close the adjustable pressure limiting (APL) valve on the system, ensuring it closes smoothly and correctly without cross-threading.
23. Perform a pressure leak test on the breathing system by occluding the patient-end tubing (using a thumb or occlusion cap) and pressing the emergency oxygen flush valve to fill the reservoir bag. (Be careful not to overfill the reservoir bag, as this could cause damage and create micro-holes.) Systems with modern APL valves may release pressure at this point; this is a safety feature of the modern systems, although the reservoir bag should still remain distended and not collapse.
24. If the system has a pressure manometer incorporated within it, fill the reservoir bag until the manometer reaches 20 cmH$_2$O.
25. Observe the bag closely and ensure it remains distended for 30 seconds, or the manometer remains at 20 cmH$_2$O.
26. Gently compress the reservoir bag (for coaxial Bain system checks see Step 27).
27. To check a co-axial Bain system:
   i. Follow steps 22 to 26.
   ii. Inspect the inner inspiratory tubing for any blockages or damage.

  iii. Set the oxygen flow at 2 litres/minute.
  iv. Briefly occlude the inner inspiratory tube using an occlusion cap (or a 2 ml syringe plunger).
  v. Back pressure from the occluded inspiratory tubing should cause the flowmeter (bobbin) to drop.
  vi. Compress the bag gently. Any leaks should be detected at this point.
28. Open the APL valve to release the pressure within the reservoir bag. *Systems with CO_2 absorbent should not have the occlusion cap removed to reduce pressure in the reservoir bag as this could force dust from the absorbent into the breathing tubing, which could be inhaled by the next patient.*
29. Check the correct operation of all valves, including unidirectional valves within a circle system, and ensure they are not sticking.
30. Check all exhaust valves for correct operation.
31. Check that the anaesthetic gas scavenging system is switched on and functioning correctly.
32. Check the scavenging tubing is attached to the appropriate exhaust port of the breathing system and the scavenging system (either active or passive).
33. Check the APL valves to ensure they are not cross-threading or sticking, and are left in an open position.

NOTES

Drugs

Commonly used opioids [3,9]

Drug	Opioid receptor effects	Analgesic efficacy
Morphine	Mu agonist	Potent analgesic agent
Methadone	Mu agonist	Equipotent to morphine
Pethidine	Mu agonist	Potent but very short-acting
Fentanyl	Mu agonist	More potent than morphine
Buprenorphine	Partial mu agonist	Significantly less potent than morphine
Butorphanol	Mu antagonist/ kappa agonist	Poor analgesic but good sedation
Naloxone	Antagonist	No analgesic properties (opioid reversal)

NOTES

Duration of action	Routes of administration	Controlled Drug status
4–6 hours	i.v. (dilute with saline and give slowly; bolus or CRI), i.m., s.c., epidural (use a preservative-free solution)	Schedule 2
4 hours	i.v., i.m., s.c. Not routinely given by CRI or epidural	Schedule 2
1–1.5 hours	i.m., s.c. Do not give i.v.	Schedule 2
20–30 minutes	i.v. (CRI or bolus)	Schedule 2
4–12 hours	i.v., i.m., s.c. (not recommended), oral, transmucosal	Schedule 3
1.5–2 hours	i.v., i.m., s.c.	Not subject to Controlled Drug Regulations
30–60 minutes	i.v.	Not subject to Controlled Drug Regulations

NOTES

Anaesthetic agents – intravenous[6]

Steroids

- **Alfaxalone**
  #### Usage and effects
  - Alfaxan contains 10 mg/ml of alfaxalone. It is available in Australia, New Zealand and the UK. Because it does not contain Cremophor EL it can be used in dogs as well as cats for the induction and maintenance of anaesthesia
  #### Contraindications and warnings
  - It must be injected slowly to avoid respiratory depression and resultant apnoea

Dissociative anaesthetic agents

Produce a light plane of anaesthesia along with profound analgesia. The animal appears dissociated from its surroundings and procedures being carried out

- **Ketamine**
  #### Usage and effects
  - Used on its own and in various combinations with alpha-2 agonists, opiate analgesics and benzodiazepines to produce anaesthesia in dogs, cats, rabbits and other exotics
  #### Contraindications and warnings
  - Not suitable for use in animals with impaired renal function or hepatic function

- **Tiletamine**
  #### Usage and effects
  - Similar to ketamine
  - Available premixed with zolazepam (a benzodiazepine) in USA and Australia

Substituted phenols

- **Propofol**
  #### Usage and effects
  - Marketed as a milky white emulsion in soya bean oil, egg phosphatide and glycerol
  - Intravenous injection results in a rapid induction of anaesthesia which, if not maintained with an inhalation agent or further boluses of propofol, lasts about 15–20 minutes
  - Rapidly metabolized in the liver and elsewhere in the body. Animals with impaired liver function are less likely to experience prolonged recoveries when given propofol
  - Because of its rapid metabolism, it is non-cumulative and can be used as a maintenance anaesthetic agent. When used for this

purpose, it is often delivered as a constant-rate infusion using a syringe driver
- Does not produce prolonged anaesthesia in Greyhounds and other sight hounds

Contraindications and warnings
- Some individuals develop severe muscle twitches after prolonged use
- Following intravenous injection, a transient fall in blood pressure and cardiac output is seen along with a brief period of apnoea
- The cardiovascular effects of propofol are at least as profound as those seen with thiopental
- Propofol's main advantage over thiopental is its short duration of action and extra-hepatic metabolism. It is not a 'safer' anaesthetic even though it is often sold to owners as such
- Most solutions do not contain preservatives but there are some available that do; thus care must be taken to adhere to disposal advice for individual products

Pharmacology of injectable agents [9]

■ Alfaxalone

Formulations, preparation and storage: Solubilized in a cyclodextrin that does not cause histamine release; can be used in cats and dogs. No preservative so should be discarded or used immediately once bottle is opened

Routes of administration: i.v., i.m.

Cardiovascular system effects: Myocardial depression associated with compensatory increase in heart rate

Respiratory system effects: Respiratory depression. May cause apnoea after injection

Comments: Recovery can be stormy if given to unpremedicated animals. Can be used to maintain anaesthesia by incremental injection or CRI

■ Ketamine

Formulations, preparation and storage: Contains preservative; does not need to be stored in the fridge

Routes of administration: i.v., i.m.

Cardiovascular system effects: Stimulates sympathetic nervous system, increases heart rate. Minimal effects on cardiac output

Respiratory system effects: Minimal effects; may cause apneustic breathing pattern

Comments: Can cause pain on i.m. injection. Only use in premedicated animals, commonly combined with a benzodiazepine. Low doses for induction; higher doses for period of anaesthesia as part of total injectable technique. Recovery can be 'spacey' or stormy, particularly in dogs. Analgesic. ➡

■ **Propofol**

Formulations, preparation and storage: Propofol solubilized in egg phosphatide and soya bean oil, with benzyl alcohol as a preservative, can be used for up to 28 days after the bottle is broached

Routes of administration: i.v. (does not cause thrombophlebitis if injected outside vein)

Cardiovascular system effects: Myocardial depression, vasodilation and bradycardia

Respiratory system effects: Respiratory depression. May cause apnoea after rapid injection

Comments: Relatively non-accumulative and can be used to maintain anaesthesia by incremental injection or CRI. The preparation containing preservative is not suitable for CRI

Anaesthetic agents – volatile[6]

■ **Isoflurane**

Usage and effects
- Less soluble than halothane and therefore produces even more rapid induction of and recovery from anaesthesia
- Can be used as both induction and maintenance agent
- Very useful for induction of anaesthesia in small mammals
- Does not sensitize heart to adrenaline as much as halothane and so causes fewer cardiac arrhythmias
- More potent respiratory depressant than halothane

Contraindications and warnings
- Produces less severe myocardial depression than halothane (but overall fall in blood pressure is similar, due to more profound peripheral vasodilation)

Minimum alveolar concentration %	Solubility coefficient (blood/gas)	Maximum legal occupational exposure limits (ppm)	Global warming potential
Dog 1.28 Cat 1.63 Rabbit 2.05	1.5	50	1100

■ **Sevoflurane**

Usage and effects
- Less soluble still than isoflurane so rapid induction of and recovery from anaesthesia as well as rapid changes in anaesthetic depth
- Depresses myocardial contractility (strength of heart's contractions) – similar to isoflurane, as is degree of peripheral vasodilation produced
- Does not sensitize heart to adrenaline so causes fewer arrhythmias

Contraindications and warnings
- Rapid recoveries from anaesthesia can expose poor analgesic techniques – animals can wake up quickly and vocalize in pain. This must not be dismissed as dysphoria or 'a reaction to the anaesthetic'
- Reacts with dry soda lime to produce 'Compound A' – a chemical known to be toxic to rats. It is not toxic to dogs in concentrations found during clinical use and sevoflurane can be used with circuits containing soda lime in dogs

Minimum alveolar concentration %	Solubility coefficient (blood/gas)	Maximum legal occupational exposure limits (ppm)	Global warming potential
Dog 2.1–2.36 Cat 2.58 Rabbit 3.7	0.68	60	1600

■ Desflurane
Usage and effects
- Very volatile (is nearly boiling at room temperature) and must be delivered using special electronically controlled vaporizer/blender
- The least soluble of all the volatile agents and so produces the most rapid induction and recovery

Contraindications and warnings
- Not yet in common use in veterinary practice

Minimum alveolar concentration %	Solubility coefficient (blood/gas)	Maximum legal occupational exposure limits (ppm)	Global warming potential
Dog 7.2 Cat 9.8 Rabbit 5.7–7.1	0.42	–	–

NOTES

Anaesthetic emergencies

How to perform CPR [10]

The guidelines for performing veterinary CPR have changed from the traditional ABC approach. The focus is now more on maintaining perfusion of tissues/organs with blood, and this can be achieved by delivering high quality chest compressions with minimal interruptions. These compressions should be delivered in uninterrupted 2-minute cycles, with patients placed in lateral recumbency in most situations. A compression rate of 100–120 per minute will achieve a compression depth of 1/3 to 1/2 the width of the chest, allowing full recall in between compressions. Early intubation is also valuable for patients ventilated at a rate of around 10 breaths per minute (to avoid hypocapnia).

1. Note the time.
2. Alert other members of staff.
3. Start compressions at approximately 100–120 beats per minute.
4. Secure the airway and start ventilation at 8–10 breaths per minute and 100% O_2. Connect to capnograph if possible.
5. Continue for at least 2 minutes.
6. Additional personnel should secure intravenous access and apply ECG and other monitoring; one person should write down all interventions.
7. Administer adrenaline and atropine if no ECG applied, asystole or pulseless electrical activity (PEA).
8. Assess for return of spontaneous circulation using ECG, stethoscope or pulse palpation.

Drugs

- Because only 25–40% of normal cardiac output is achieved using chest compressions alone, drugs play a vital role in CPR. Vasopressors, e.g. adrenaline, are an essential part of the CPR drug protocol.
- Provided that cardiac massage is achieving good cardiac output, intravenous injection (central or peripheral) is the best route of administration of emergency drugs.

- If venous access is not possible, the intraosseous or intratracheal route may be used.
- Intracardiac administration of emergency drugs is now contraindicated.

For more information on the latest veterinary CPR guidelines see **www.acvecc-recover.org**

Contents and use of an anaesthetic emergency box[1]

- Pressure bag for rapid fluid infusion
- 50% dextrose
- Lactated Ringer's solution
- Ambu bag
- Endotracheal (ET) tubes, various sizes
- Laryngoscope
- Hypodermic needles, various sizes
- Assorted intravenous catheters
- Gauze sponges/swabs
- 25 mm wide adhesive tape
- 50 mm roll of gauze
- Polyethylene urinary catheters
- Suture materials
- 3-way taps
- Thoracostomy tray
- Clippers
- 4% chlorhexidine gluconate or 10% povidone–iodine
- 70% surgical spirit
- Electrocardiogram monitor, leads, clips and conduction gel
- Doppler blood pressure monitor
- Defibrillator
- Drugs (see table over)

➥

Drug	Indications	Dosage
Adrenaline	Severe bradycardia Ventricular fibrillation Ventricular asystole Pulseless electrical activity	0.01–0.2 mg/kg i.v. bolus q3–5min 0.04–0.4 mg/kg intratracheal 0.1–1 µg/kg/min i.v. CRI
Atropine sulphate	Sinus bradycardia Atrioventricular block Ventricular asystole	0.04 mg/kg i.v 0.4 mg/kg intratracheal
Calcium gluconate (10%)	Hyperkalaemia Hypocalcaemia Calcium channel-blocker toxicity Hypermagnesaemia	0.5–1.0 ml/kg i.v. to effect; closely observe the ECG
Diltiazem	Supraventricular tachycardia Ventricular fibrillation Hypertrophic cardiomyopathy	0.25 mg/kg i.v. bolus, to cumulative dose of 0.75 mg/kg
Dobutamine	Myocardial failure Low cardiac output	5–20 µg/kg/min CRI
Dopamine	Bradycardia Low cardiac output Hypotension	5–10 µg/kg/min CRI for increased contractility and cardiac output 10–20 µg/kg/min CRI for vasoconstriction
Furosemide	Cerebral/pulmonary oedema Congestive heart failure Hypertension Oliguria/anuria	Dogs: 2–4 mg/kg i.v., i.m. Cats: 1–2 mg/kg i.v., i.m.
Lidocaine	Ventricular tachycardia Ventricular fibrillation	Dogs: 2–8 mg/kg i.v. bolus followed by 30–80 µg/kg/min CRI Cats: 0.25–0.5 mg/kg i.v. bolus followed by 10–20 µg/kg/min CRI
Mannitol	Cerebral oedema Oliguria	0.5–1.0 mg/kg i.v. given slowly over 10 min
Morphine sulphate	Analgesia/sedation Vasodilator Pulmonary oedema	0.04–0.08 mg/kg i.v., i.m., s.c.
Naloxone	Electromechanical dissociation Narcotic overdose	0.015–0.04 mg/kg i.v., i.m., s.c., intratracheal (give to effect)
Sodium bicarbonate	Severe metabolic acidosis	0.5–1.0 mEq/kg i.v.

NOTES

NOTES

Cleaning and sterilization

Cleaning the operating theatre[6]

Daily cleaning

All horizontal surfaces, lights, furniture and equipment should be damp-dusted daily with a suitable disinfectant that is bactericidal, fungicidal, sporicidal and virucidal. The disinfectant should be diluted according to the manufacturer's instructions and handled only when wearing disposable plastic apron, gloves and mask.

As soon as the patient has been removed from theatre and before the next one arrives in the anaesthetic room:

- Remove dirty instruments and place in cool water and cleaning solution for later cleaning and re-sterilization
- Wipe over all flat surfaces, anaesthetic equipment, operating table and other equipment that may have become dirty, using a suitable disinfectant
- Clean the floor only if necessary (usually this applies only to the soiled areas around the operating table)
- Reposition the table, heating pad and diathermy plate
- Restock if necessary
- Prepare the instruments and equipment for the next surgery
- Place waste materials in the appropriate receptacles.

Immediately after surgery finishes at the end of the day, the operating room should be cleaned thoroughly. This is best done at the end of the day when no further operations are scheduled. This gives any airborne particles, disturbed during cleaning, time to settle before the next procedure begins. At the end of the day the operating room should be ready for use again, either for the following day or in case of any emergencies.

- Clean and re-sterilize all instruments that have been used during the day, ready for use again when needed.
- Thoroughly clean all surfaces, equipment and the floor within theatre, including the scrub sink area.
- Restock and refill supplies and drugs as necessary.
- Empty and clean all bins and vacuum cleaners.
- Wash all drapes and theatre clothing, including boots and shoes worn in theatre.

Weekly cleaning

Weekly cleaning is important to maintain the standards of cleanliness and reach all areas not cleaned in the daily routine. This cleaning should include the preparation rooms and changing rooms associated with the theatre.

- The operating room should be emptied of movable equipment, which should be cleaned (including the castors, where appropriate) before it is returned to theatre.
- Working from ceiling to floor, all fixed structures should be cleaned – including all walls, floors, scrub sinks and drains.
- Although cupboards are not recommended in theatre, they are necessary in the preparation and scrub area; all of them should be emptied, cleaned and restocked during the weekly clean.
- Clean removable filters on items such as suction machines and forced air-warming devices (e.g. Bairhuggers).

Folding a gown[9]

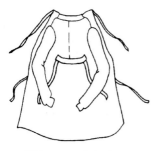

(a) Lay gown flat out.

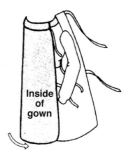

(b) Fold side to middle.

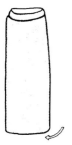

(c) Fold over other side to edge.

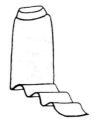

(d) Concertina lengthways.

(e) Pick up by inside of collar after autoclaving.

NOTES

Folding a surgical drape⁹

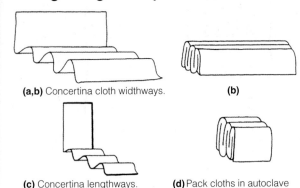

(a,b) Concertina cloth widthways.

(b)

(c) Concertina lengthways.

(d) Pack cloths in autoclave drum or autoclave bags sealed with indicating tape.

Folding a plain drape⁹

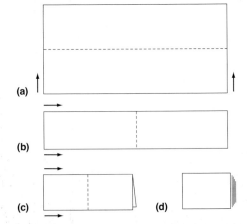

(a)

(b)

(c)

(d)

Folding a plain drape, corner to corner: **(a)** The drape is folded in half widthways, and then **(b–d)** folded in half lengthways three times, so that there are two corners at the top.

Packing instruments for sterilization[6]

- ■ **Linen drapes**
  - **Advantages:** Readily available; conforming; can be used to pack difficult items
  - **Disadvantages:** Porous; liable to wear; time spent laundering and folding
  - **Type of sterilization method:** Autoclave with drying cycle or ethylene oxide if not too tightly packed

- ■ **Paper drapes**
  - **Advantages:** Water-resistant so useful as outer layer to package surgical kits
  - **Disadvantages:** Non-conforming; can be torn easily
  - **Type of sterilization method:** Autoclave with drying cycle or ethylene oxide

- ■ **Self-seal sterilization bags**
  - **Advantages:** Easy to pack; clear front so able to see contents
  - **Disadvantages:** Heavier or sharp instruments may puncture bag (to prevent punctures double packing may be necessary, which increases cost)
  - **Type of sterilization method:** Autoclave with ethylene oxide

- ■ **Nylon films**
  - **Advantages:** Cheap; long-lasting; readily available
  - **Disadvantages:** Punctures easily – punctures not easily seen so may be missed
  - **Type of sterilization method:** Autoclave

- ■ **Metal tins**
  - **Advantages:** Easy to pack; very long lasting after initial expense; cannot be punctured by sharp or heavy instruments
  - **Disadvantages:** Expensive to buy; bulky to store; need a large autoclave with a drying cycle
  - **Type of sterilization method:** Autoclave or hot-air oven

- ■ **Special polythene bags supplied by manufacturers of ethylene oxide**
  - **Advantages:** Easy to use, strong bags
  - **Disadvantages:** Must use specific polythene bags with correct equipment; can over pack so gas cannot circulate
  - **Type of sterilization method:** Ethylene oxide

- ■ **Cardboard cartons**
  - **Advantages:** Sturdy and not easily punctured by sharp objects; regular shape makes them neat to store
  - **Disadvantages:** Expensive to buy; can be bulky to store
  - **Type of sterilization method:** Autoclave with drying cycle

NOTES

Indicators of sterilization[6]

Method	Comments	Use with
Chemical indicator strips	Show a colour change when exposed to the correct conditions. Should be placed in centre of pack before sterilization	
	■ Chemical indicator strips: paper strips that change colour when exposed to correct conditions of temperature, pressure and time; also available for ethylene oxide	Autoclave, ethylene oxide
	■ Browne's tube: small glass tube filled with orange liquid that changes to green when correct temperature is reached and maintained for correct length of time. Available for different temperatures	Autoclave, hot-air oven
Indicator tape	Often used as method of securing other packing methods. Both of these tapes only indicate exposure, not that correct time or pressure has been achieved; therefore cannot be considered as reliable method for checking sterilization	
	■ Bowie Dick tape: beige with series of lines on it that change to black after exposure to temperature of 121°C	Autoclave
	■ Ethylene oxide tape: green with series of lines that change to red after exposure to EO gas	Ethylene oxide
Spore strips	Paper strips that contain a controlled-count spore population. After sterilization, strips are cultured for 72 hours to see if all spores destroyed. Main disadvantage is delay in obtaining results	Autoclave, hot-air oven, ethylene oxide

NOTES

Gowning and gloving

Putting on a surgical gown[9]

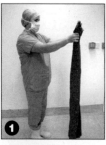
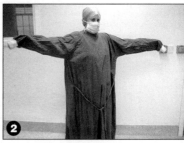
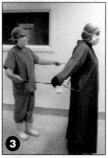
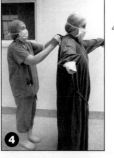

1. The sterile gown (folded inside out) is taken from its sterile pack, held at the shoulders and allowed to fall open.
2. One hand is slipped into each sleeve. No attempt should be made to try to pull the sleeves over the shoulder or to readjust the gown, as this will lead to contamination of the hands or outside of the gown.
3. An unscrubbed assistant should pull the back of the gown over the shoulders (touching only the inside surface of the gown) and secure the ties at the back.
4. With the hands retained within the sleeves, the waist ties should be picked up and held out to the sides. In the case of a **back-tying gown**, the unscrubbed assistant will then take the ends of the waist ties and secure them at the back. The back of the gown is now no longer sterile and must not come into contact with sterile equipment, drapes and gowns.

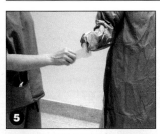

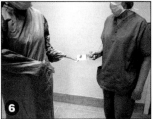

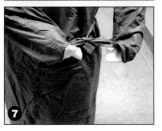

5. In the case of a **side-tying gown**, the unscrubbed assistant takes hold of the paper tape on the longer waist tape and takes the tie around the back to the opposite side.

6. The scrubbed person then pulls the tape, so that the paper tape comes away.

7. The gown is tied at the waist by the scrubbed person. This type of gown provides an all-round sterile field.

NOTES

Closed gloving procedure[9]

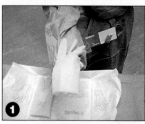

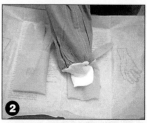

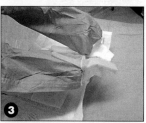

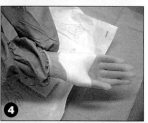

1. Hands remain within the sleeves of the gown. The glove packet is turned so that the fingers point towards the body. (The right glove will now be on the left and *vice versa*.)
2. The glove is picked up at the rim of the cuff of the glove.
3. The hand is turned over so that the glove lies on the palm surface with fingers of the glove still pointing towards the body.
4. The rim is picked up with the opposite hand.

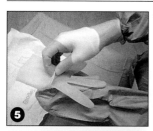

5. It is then pulled over the fingers and over the dorsal surface of the wrist.
6. The glove is then pulled on as the fingers are pushed forwards.

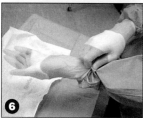

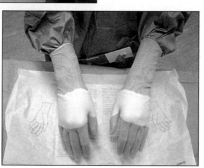

NOTES

Open gloving procedure[9]

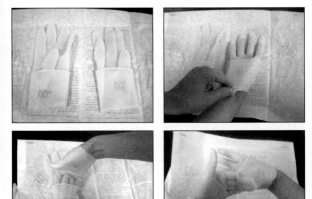

1. The glove pack is opened by an assistant.
2. With the left hand, the right glove is picked up by the turned-down cuff, holding only the inner surface of the glove.
3. The glove is pulled on to the right hand. Do not unfold the cuff at this stage.
4. The gloved fingers of the right hand are placed under the cuff of the left glove and pulled on to the left hand, holding only the outer surface of this glove.
5. The rim of the left glove is hooked over the thumb whilst the cuff of the gown (if worn) is adjusted.
6. The cuff of the left glove is pulled over the cuff of the gown (if worn) using the fingers of the right hand.
7. The final steps are then repeated for the right hand.

Scrubbing

Surgical scrub solutions[9]

Agent	Properties
Povidone–iodine	■ Iodine combined with a detergent ■ Broad-spectrum antimicrobial activity (bactericidal, virucidal and fungicidal) ■ May cause severe skin reactions and irritation in some individuals ■ Efficacy impaired by organic matter
Chlorhexidine	■ Effective against many bacteria (including *Escherichia coli* and *Pseudomonas* spp.) ■ Virucidal, fungicidal and sporicidal properties ■ Effective level of activity in presence of organic material ■ Longer residual activity than povidone–iodine ■ Relatively low toxicity to tissue
Triclosan	■ Newer agent, claimed to be antibacterial against both Gram-positive and Gram-negative bacteria

Skin preparation technique[9]

1. Put on surgical gloves, to prevent contamination of the patient's skin from your hands. It is not necessary, however, for the gloves to be sterile during the initial preparation.
2. Using lint-free swabs, a surgical scrub solution and a little warm water, clean the site. There are 2 options for how this can be achieved:
   – Concentric circles: begin at the proposed incision site and work outwards.
   – Back-and-forth: clean the whole clipped surgical site, then focus on the proposed incision site using a back-and-forth action.
   Once the edges of the clipped area are reached, discard the swab and take a new one.
3. Continue this procedure until the area is clean, i.e. there is no discoloration or dirt visible on a white swab.
4. Avoid over-wetting the patient. For limb surgery that does not involve the foot, it should be wrapped in a non-sterile ➡

cohesive bandage to allow for draping once transferred into the operating theatre. Care should be taken to avoid soaking the coat, as this will increase the risk of 'strike-through' from the drapes, should material drapes be used, and may make the patient hypothermic, especially in the case of small pets.

5. Move the patient into the theatre and position it for surgery. For limb surgery, a limb tie or tape is applied over the bandaged foot and attached to a transfusion stand. This allows preparation around all sides of the limb as the limb is suspended.

6. As the site is likely to have been contaminated to some extent in the transition to the theatre, clean the skin again in the manner previously described. Sterile gloves, saline and swabs are sometimes used, although this is not always necessary. Lint-free swabs should always be used, and never cotton wool, to prevent any residue being left on the skin.

7. The final stage of preparation involves application of an antiseptic skin solution that can ideally be sprayed over the surgical site and allowed to dry on to the skin, e.g. chlorhexidine isopropyl.

Scrub routine[9]

1. Remove watch and jewellery.
2. Adjust the water supply (which should be elbow- or foot-operated) to a suitable temperature and flow.
3. Wash the hands thoroughly using an antimicrobial soap, adopting a good hand washing technique. At this stage, clean the nails using a nail pick.
4. Once the hands have been washed, wash the arms up to the elbows. Always keep the hands higher than the elbows so that water drains down towards the unscrubbed upper arms. The purpose of this stage of the procedure is to remove organic matter and grease from the skin.
5. Rinse the hands and then the lower arms, allowing water to wash away the soap from the hands towards the elbows.
6. Using a surgical scrub solution begin the surgical scrub.

Use only sufficient water to produce a lather, as bactericidal properties of the scrub solution are dependent on contact time with the skin. Excessive amounts of water will rinse away the scrub solution before it has achieved its aim.

7. Lather the surgical scrub solution over the arms before scrubbing the hands. Take a sterile scrubbing brush and systematically scrub the hands. Scrub the palms of the hand, wrist and four surfaces of each finger and thumb (back, front and both sides) and the nails. Either rinse the brush and use it on the other hand or discard it and take a second brush. It is not recommended that the backs of the hands and arms are scrubbed as this may lead to excoriation, which predisposes to infection.

8. When both hands have been scrubbed for the correct contact time, drop the brush into the sink. Begin to rinse the hands and arms as before, ensuring that the hands are constantly kept above the elbows to allow the water to drain away from the hands and off the elbows.

9. The final stage is to wash the hands and wrists in surgical scrub solution. This time the scrubbing process is not extended to the elbow, so that there is no danger that a previously unscrubbed area is touched.

10. Rinse the hands and arms as before.

11. Take a sterile hand towel, holding it at arm's length. Use a different quarter to dry each hand and each arm. Then discard the hand towel.

Once the scrubbing up routine has started, the hands must not touch the taps, sink or scrub dispenser. If these are inadvertently touched, the process must start again at Step 3.

Sutures

Absorbable suture materials[6]

Suture material	Trade names	Mono/ multifilament	Synthetic/ natural
Polyglactin 910	Vicryl (Ethicon) Polysorb (USSC)	Multi (braided)	Synthetic
Polydioxanone	PDS II (Ethicon)	Mono	Synthetic
Polyglycolic acid	Dexon (USSC)	Multi	Synthetic
Poliglecaprone 25	Monocryl (Ethicon) Caprosyn (USSC)	Mono	Synthetic

Coated	Duration of strength	Absorption	Comments/uses
Yes (calcium stearate)	Retains 50% of tensile strength at 14 days, 20% at 21 days	Absorption 60–90 days by hydrolysis	Dyed or undyed Low tissue reactivity Uses: subcutis, muscle, eyes, hollow viscera
No	Retains 70% tensile strength at 14 days, 14% at 56 days	Only minimal absorption by 90 days, absorbed by 180 days Absorbed by hydrolysis	Good for infected sites as monofilament Very strong but springy Minimal tissue reaction Uses: subcutis, muscle, sometimes eyes
Can be coated with polymers	Retains 20% at 14 days	Complete absorption by 100–120 days Absorbed by hydrolysis	Similar to polyglactin but has considerable tissue drag Uses: as for polyglactin.
No	Retains approximately 60% at 7 days, 30% at 14 days Wound support maintained for 20 days	Complete absorption between 90 and 120 days Absorbed by hydrolysis	New synthetic suture material Less springy than other monofilament absorbables with minimal tissue reaction and drag Available dyed or undyed

Non-absorbable suture materials[6]

Suture material	Trade names	Mono- or multifilament	Synthetic/natural
Polyamide (nylon)	Ethilon (Ethicon), Monosof (USSC)	Mono	Synthetic
Polybutester	Novafil (Davis & Geck)	Mono	Synthetic
Polypropylene	Prolene (Ethicon), Surgipro (USSC)	Mono	Synthetic
Braided silk	Mersilk (Ethicon)	Multi	Natural
Braided polyamide	Supramid or Nurolon (Ethicon)	Multi	Synthetic
Surgical stainless steel wire		Available as either mono or multi	Synthetic

Coated	Knot security	Duration	Comments/uses
No	Fair	Permanent	Causes minimal tissue reaction and has little tissue drag
No	Fair	Permanent	Very similar to Ethilon, with similar properties
No	Fair, can produce bulky knots that untie easily	Permanent	Very inert, produces only minimal tissue reaction Very strong but also very springy Little tissue drag
Wax coat	Excellent	Eventually may fragment and break down	Natural material with good handling properties but high tissue reactivity and should not be used in infected sites
Encased in outer sheath	Good	Outer sheath can be broken	Better handling characteristics than monofilament polyamide Can be used in the skin but should not be used as buried suture
No	Excellent but knots may be difficult to tie	Permanent	Not commonly used now but can be useful in bone or tendon Difficult to handle, may break

Summary of suture patterns[6]

Continuous

- **Simple continuous (SC)**
  - **Description:** Running stitch
  - **Particular features:** Rapidly placed; prone to patient interference if used in skin; theoretically insecure
  - **Typical application:** Fascia, including midline; muscle; viscera

- **Intradermal/subcuticular**
  - **Description:** Buried continuous stitch to close skin
  - **Particular features:** Slower than other skin patterns; resists tension; avoids patient interference; does not require removal
  - **Typical application:** Skin; presence of tension; sites prone to interference (e.g. castration)

Interrupted

- **Simple interrupted appositional (SIA)**
  - **Description:** Individual stitches placed as simple loops across wound
  - **Particular features:** The standard pattern; produces good apposition
  - **Typical application:** Skin closure; midline closure; viscera closure

- **Horizontal mattress**
  - **Description:** Placed as loops with a bite on each side of wound parallel to wound edge
  - **Particular features:** Produces some eversion; resists effects of tension more than SIA
  - **Typical application:** Skin, especially in presence of tension

- **Cruciate mattress**
  - **Description:** Similar to horizontal mattress but strands cross over wound
  - **Particular features:** Less eversion than above; resists effects of tension more than SIA; faster than above
  - **Typical application:** Skin, especially in presence of tension

- **Vertical mattress**
  - **Description:** Placed as loops with a bite on each side of wound perpendicular to wound edge
  - **Particular features:** Produces some eversion; resists effects of tension more than SIA; interferes with blood supply less than horizontal mattress
  - **Typical application:** Skin, especially in presence of tension; most commonly used interspersed with SIA to resist effects of tension

NOTES

NOTES

References

1. *BSAVA Guide to Procedures in Small Animal Practice* (2010), ed. N. Bexfield and K. Lee

2. *BSAVA Manual of Canine and Feline Advanced Veterinary Nursing, 2nd edn* (2008), ed. A. Hotson Moore and S. Rudd

3. *BSAVA Manual of Canine and Feline Anaesthesia and Analgesia, 2nd edn* (2007), ed. C. Seymour and T. Duke-Novakovski

4. *BSAVA Manual of Canine and Feline Cardiorespiratory Medicine, 2nd edn* (2010), ed. V. Luis Fuentes, L.R. Johnson and S. Dennis

5. *BSAVA Manual of Canine and Feline Emergency and Critical Care, 2nd edn* (2007), ed. L.G. King and A. Boag

6. *BSAVA Manual of Practical Veterinary Nursing* (2007), ed. E. Mullineaux and M. Jones

7. *BSAVA Manual of Small Animal Practice Management and Development* (2012), ed. C. Clarke and M. Chapman

8. *BSAVA Pocketbook for Vets* (2012) ed. S. Middleton

9. *BSAVA Textbook of Veterinary Nursing, 5th edn* (2011), ed. B. Cooper, E. Mullineaux and L. Turner

10. Written by Louise O'Dwyer

Index

Abdominal bandage 66

Absorbable suture materials 170–1

Adverse reactions to blood transfusions 93–4

Anaesthesia and analgesia

    drugs 144–9

    emergencies

        CPR 150–1

        emergency box 151–2

    equipment

        breathing circuits 130–7

        checks 141–3

        fresh gas flow rates 139–40

    risk, ASA scale 129

Arterial blood sampling 31–3

ASA scale of anaesthetic risk 129

Bandaging

    abdominal bandage 66

    ear and head bandage 64

    Ehmer sling 69

    foot and lower limb bandage 67

    Robert Jones bandage 62–3

    tail bandage 70

    thoracic bandage 65

    Velpeau sling 68

Biochemistry reference ranges 43

Blood

    biochemistry/haematology reference ranges 43

    loss calculation 79–80

    pressure

        direct measurement 12

        indirect measurement 12

        values 16

sampling
    arterial 31–3
    venous 34–8
smear preparation 40–2
staining procedures 42–3
transfusion
    administering the blood 90–3
    adverse reactions 93–4
    blood typing 89–90
    calculating blood loss 79–80
    collection 80–5
    cross-matching 85–8
Body Condition System
    cats 10–11
    dogs 8–9
Body temperature 1
Breathing circuits 130–7

Catheter management 22
Cleaning the operating theatre 155–6
Closed gloving procedure 164–5
Coat brushing 46–7
Colloid solutions 78
CPR 150–1
Cross-matching blood 85–8
Crystalloid solutions 78

Dehydration, clinical signs 75
Drains, management 71
Dressings *see* Wound dressings

Ear and head bandage 64
ECG 16
Ehmer sling 69
Electrocardiography 16
Emergency box, anaesthetic 151–2

➡

Faecal examinations 45
Feeding tubes
    nursing considerations 24
    selection 23
Film faults 125–6
Fine needle aspiration 50, 51–2
Fluid therapy
    calculating fluid loss 76
    calculating fluid rates 77
    colloid solutions 78
    crystalloid solutions 78
    dehydration, clinical signs 75
Folding
    gowns 157
    plain drapes 158
    surgical drapes 158
Foot and lower limb bandage 67

Gas flow rates 139–40
Gloving
    closed 164–5
    open 166
Gown
    folding 157
    putting on 162–3

Haematology reference ranges 43
Hair and skin sampling
    coat brushing 46–7
    fine needle aspiration 50
    hair plucking 48–9
    hand-held lens examination 46
    impression smears 50
    Mackenzie brush 47
    skin biopsy 50–1
    skin scraping 47–8
    sticky tape preparation 49–50

Hawksley reader, PCV determination 39
Heart rate 1
Humphrey ADE circuit 136–7
Humphrey APL valve 137–9

Imaging
    film faults 125–6
    see also Radiographic positioning
Impression smears 50
Inpatient care 21–27
Instruments, packing for sterilization 159
Intravenous catheter management 22

Laboratory
    blood 31–43
    faecal examinations 45
    fine needle aspiration 51–2
    hair and skin sampling 46–51
    packaging laboratory samples for external analysis 53–4
    urine 44

Mackenzie brush sampling 47
Massage 25
Mucous membrane colour 5

Non-absorbable suture materials 172–3
Nutritional assessment 7

Open gloving procedure 166
Operating theatre *see* Theatre

Packaging laboratory samples 53–4
Pain
    assessment 6–7
    behavioural indicators 6
    scales 7
PCV determination 39
Physiotherapy 24–7

Radiographic positioning
    abdomen 118–19
    forelimbs 102–6, 121–2, 124–5
    hindlimbs 98–102, 123–4
    pelvis 97–98
    pharynx 116–17
    skull 107–12, 119–21
    spine 113–16
    thorax 117–18
Recumbent patients 21
Respiratory rate 1
Resting energy requirement (RER) 23
Robert Jones bandage 62–3

Scrubbing
    scrub routine 168–9
    skin preparation technique 167–8
    surgical scrub solutions 167
Skin
    aseptic preparation 167–8
    biopsy 50–1
    sampling *see* Hair and skin sampling
Squash preparation 52
Staining procedures 42–3
Sterilization
    indicators 161
    packing instruments 159
Sticky tape skin preparation 49–50
Surgical drape
    folding 158
    sterilization 159
Surgical scrub solutions 167
Sutures
    absorbable suture materials 170–1
    non-absorbable suture materials 172–3
    summary of suture patterns 174

Tail bandage 70
Theatre
    cleaning and sterilization 155–61
    gowning and gloving 162–6
    scrubbing 167–9
    sutures 170–4
Thoracic bandage 65
Triage and emergency care
    blood transfusion 79–94
    fluid therapy 75–8
Typing, blood 89–90

Urinalysis 44
Urinary catheters, cleaning 22
Urine specific gravity (USG) 44

Velpeau sling 68
Venous blood sampling 34–8
Vital signs 1

Wood's lamp 46
Wound drains 71
Wound dressings
    dry 57–8
    interactive 58–61
    topical 61

Emergency doses
for dogs and cats

ALWAYS read the relevant monographs.

Cardiac emergencies
- **Asystole or pulseless electrical activity**
  - Adrenaline: 20 μg (micrograms)/kg i.v. – this is equivalent to 1 ml/5 kg using 1:10,000 concentration (100 μg/ml). Double dose if used intratracheally.
- **Hyperkalaemic myocardial toxicity**
  - Calcium: 50–150 mg/kg calcium (boro)gluconate = 0.5–1.5 ml/kg of a 10% solution i.v. over 20–30 min *or* Soluble insulin: 0.5 IU/kg i.v. followed by 2–3 g of dextrose/unit of insulin (for urinary tract obstruction but not hypoadrenocorticism). Half the dextrose should be given as a bolus and the remainder administered i.v. over 4–6 hours.
- **Other bradyarrhythmias**
  - Atropine: 0.01–0.03 mg/kg i.v. – this is equivalent to 0.3–1 ml/20 kg using 0.6 mg/ml solution.
- **Ventricular tachycardia**
  - Lidocaine:
    Dogs: 2–8 mg/kg i.v. in 2 mg/kg boluses, followed by a constant rate i.v. infusion of 0.025–0.1 mg/kg/min.
    Cats: 0.25–2.0 mg/kg i.v. slowly in 0.25–0.5 mg/kg boluses followed by a constant rate i.v. infusion of 0.01–0.04 mg/kg/min.

Pulmonary emergencies
- **Respiratory arrest**
  - Doxapram: 5–10 mg/kg i.v., repeat according to need; duration of effect is approximately 15–20 min.
    Neonates: 1–2 drops under the tongue (oral solution) or 0.1 ml i.v. into the umbilical vein; this should be used only once.